AF392724

Controlled Release Technologies: Old and New Prospective

Controlled Release Technologies: Old and New Prospective

Muhammad Yasir Ali, PhD

Saeed Ahmed, PhD

Nisar-ur-Rahman, PhD

Published by

Muhammad Yasir Ali, Faculty of Pharmaceutical Sciences, GC University Faisalabad, Allama Iqbal Road, Punjab, 38000, Pakistan

First Edition: 2021

ISBN: 978-969-2265-00-3 (EBook)

ISBN: 978-969-2265-01-0 (Paper Back)

WORDS OF EDITOR

The history of pharmaceuticals is as old as humans are. Traditional practitioners had used drugs in one or another form in ancient times. Then came the era of traditional dosage forms including the most common and famous dosage forms e.g. tablets, capsules, syrups, etc. These dosage forms were unable to deal with the prolonged effect required, especially, when multiple frequencies of a single drug were required in a day. This originated the concept of digging new areas in the vast field of pharmaceutics. Therefore, an idea to fabricate controlled release dosage forms went through one's head. This was a paradigm change in the arena of pharmaceutical technology from conventional to controlled release formulations.

Controlled release systems are one of the powerful tools used in advanced drug delivery systems. There are different technologies used to prepare controlled release systems. Polymeric matrices, ion-exchange systems, and osmotically controlled systems are a few examples of sustained-release systems. These systems along with some more technical floating systems have been discussed here in this book, keeping pharmacy students new in the arena. Therefore, this book will accomplish the thirst of students and researchers.

Muhammad Yasir Ali
19-02-2021

CONTRIBUTORS

Arooj Khalid

Department of Pharmaceutics

GC University Faisalabad

Faisalabad

Daulat Haleem Khan, Ph.D.

Head of Department of Pharmacy

Lahore College of Pharmaceutical Sciences

Lahore

Ghulam Abbas, Ph.D.

Assistant Professor

Department of Pharmaceutics

GC University Faisalabad

Faisalabad

Muhammad Yasir Ali, Ph.D.

Assistant Professor

Department of Pharmaceutics

GC University Faisalabad

Faisalabad

Nisar-ur-Rahman, Ph.D.

Formerly, Professor of Department of Pharmacy

COMSATS University

Abbottabad

Romna Tul Janat

Department of Pharmaceutics

GC University Faisalabad

Faisalabad

Saeed Ahmad, Ph.D.

Professor and Chairman of Department of Pharmaceutical Chemistry

The Islamia University of Bahawalpur

Bahawalpur

Shahid Shah, Ph.D.

Assistant Professor

Faculty of Pharmaceutical

GC University Faisalabad

Faisalabad

DEDICATION

To my Parents

LIST OF ABBREVIATIONS

ATL	Atenolol
CA	Citric Acid
CDL	Carvedilol
CPTL	Captopril
CR	Controlled Release
CS	Chitosan
DCM	Dichloromethane
DCM	Dichloromethane
DCP	Dicalcium Phosphate
DLS	Differential Light Scattering
DMSO	Dimethyl Sulfoxide
DSC	Differential Scanning Calorimetry
EC	Ethylcellulose
EE	Entrapment Efficiency
EOP	Elementary Osmotic Pump
FDDS	Floating Drug Delivery Systems
FTIR	Fourier Transform Infrared

GI	Gastrointestinal
GIT	Gastrointestinal Tract
GRT	Gastric Retention Time
HEC	Hydroxyethyl Cellulose
HPC	Hydroxylpropyl Cellulose
HPMC	Hydroxypropyl Methylcellulose
IER	Ion-Exchange Resins
IPA	Isopropyl Alcohol
MC	Methyl Cellulose
MCG	Methylcellulose Glutarate
MCC	Microcrystalline Cellulose
MMC	Migrating Myoelectric Complex
NFDN	Nifedipine
PPOP	Push-Pull Osmotic Pump
PVA	Polyvinyl Alcohol
PVP	Polyvinylpyrrolidone
RPE	Reverse Phase Evaporation
SA	Stearylamine

SCMC	Sodium Carboxy Methylcellulose
TEM	Transmission Electron Microscopy
TFH	Thin Film Hydration Technique

CONTENTS

1. CONTROLLED RELEASE SYSTEMS

Muhammad Yasir Ali

1.1 Background

During the past three decades, significant advances have been made in the arena of controlled drug delivery due to the advancement in the fields of biopharmaceutics, pharmacokinetics, and pharmacodynamics. Normally in a typical therapeutic regimen, the drug dose and the dosing interval are controlled (Figure 1.1) so that drug concentration in the body is maintained and fewer chances of side effects along with a high level of efficacy and patient counseling are accomplished (Jain, 2003; Prajapati, et al., 2011).

Controlled release (CR) may be defined as a technique or approach by which active chemicals are made available to a specified target at a rate and duration to accomplish an intended effect. More specifically, an oral CR drug delivery system is a device or dosage form that controls the drug release into the absorption site in the GIT. It controls the drug absorption rate to achieve the desired plasma profiles defined by the steady-state pharmacology.

Oral CR drug delivery systems provide continuous delivery of drugs at predictable and reproducible kinetics for a predetermined period during gastrointestinal (GI) transit. The potential advantages of these systems are fabrication of nearly all drugs, reduced dosage frequency and total dose, decreased occurrence and intensity of toxicity, and a constant therapeutic effect (Guru, et al., 2001; Colombo, et al.,1990).

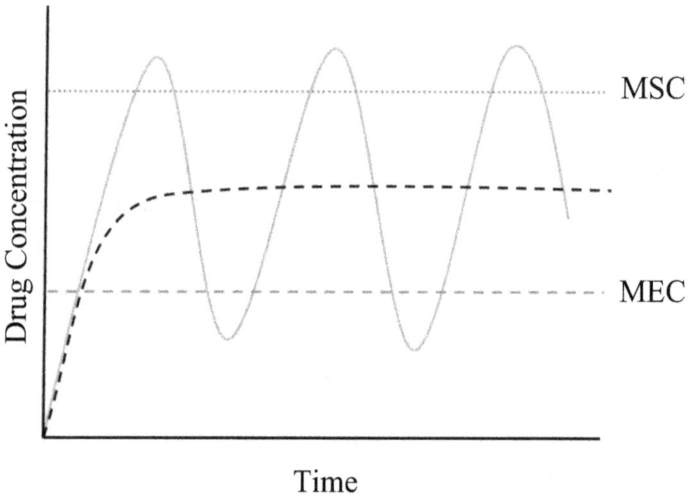

Figure 1.1: Blood concentration profiles of conventional (complete line) and controlled release systems (dotted line), after repeated drug administration (MSC: maximum safe concentration; MEC: minimum effective concentration).

Ideally, the ultimate criterion for a CR tablet is to achieve a blood level of the drug comparable to that of a liquid product administered every 4 hr. To this end, prolonged-release dosage forms are designed to release the drug to provide a drug level within the therapeutic range for 8 to 12 hr with a single dose rather than a dose every 4 hr (Boyd, et al., 2006; Herbert, et al., 2003).

Generally, the primary objectives of controlled drug delivery are to ensure safety and to improve the efficacy of drugs as well as patient compliance, which can be achieved by better control of plasma drug levels and less frequent dosing. The most convenient way to achieve CR of active agent involves a physical blending of drug with polymer matrix, followed by direct compression, compression molding, injection molding, extrusion, or solvent casting which results either in a monolithic device or in a swellable hydrogel matrix. For any controlled-release dosage form, it is very important to use a minimum number of excipients with minimum processing steps to reduce the batch-to-batch variations. When taken as an aggregate, the directly blended or single-step fabrication is the demand of today's fast going era with both a scientific and economic appeal. Since the cost of synthesizing a new polymeric substance and testing for its safety is enormous (Jolly, et al., 2008).

1.2 Advantages of Controlled Release Systems

Controlled release systems have changed the face of the pharmaceutical industry and health care setups, due to the following advantages (Saikia, et al., 2015; Ghandhi, et al., 2014);

a) Decreased GIT irritation: due to controlled drug delivery.
b) Decreased dose size: due to sustained release of the drug.
c) Decreased dosage frequency: due to extended-release of the drug.
d) Better patient compliance: due to less frequency.
e) Decrease healthcare cost: due to decreased frequency.
f) Steady plasma levels: due to predefined release pattern.
g) Improved efficacy: due to steady plasma concentrations.

1.3 Disadvantages of Controlled Release Systems

Controlled release systems also present some disadvantages as follows;

a) Dose dumping: due to system collapses.
b) Additional patient education problem: due to special instructions required in some cases.

c) Complex manufacturing process: due to increased number of formulation and processing variables.

d) The high cost of production: due to multiple steps and excipients involved.

e) Stability concerns are increased: due to the increased number of excipients.

f) Decrease retrieval of the drug: due to complex architecture.

1.4 Feasibility Assessment of Drugs

The selection of drugs suitable for the preparation of CR systems is a crucial step. There are many factors involved in the selection of drugs. These factors and drug-related properties should be kept in mind before the fabrication of such systems.

1.4.1 Solubility

Different sorts of mechanisms are present for the absorption of the drug through membranes of biological systems. These range from passive to the carrier-mediated transport mechanism. Aqueous solubility is one of the key factors influencing drug release and then its absorption through biological membranes. Non-polar drugs (most of the drugs are weak acids or bases, since their unchanged form) are preferentially permeated across lipid membranes. However, we well know that biological fluids are aqueous bases in nature so there is a question mark for the partition of such non-polar or unionized drugs between the polymeric systems in the aqueous medium. Therefore these kinds of drugs are having a self-sustained effect for absorption; controlled by partitioning. More soluble drugs are the best candidate for CR or modified release preparations. The lower limit on solubility for such product has been reported 0.1mg/ml (Sahilhusen, et al., 2014; Garg, et al., 2013; Varma, et al., 2004).

1.4.2 Dose/ Frequency

If an oral product has a dose size greater than 0.5 gm it is a poor candidate for a sustained-release system, Since the addition of sustaining dose and possibly the sustaining mechanism will, in most cases generates a substantial volume product that unacceptably large. Along with this drugs having fewer frequencies of administration are the poor candidate for modified release preparations (Kakar, et al., 2013; Sood, et al., 2003).

1.4.3 Drug Stability

Orally administered drugs can be subject to both acid-base hydrolysis and enzymatic degradation. Degradation will proceed at a reduced rate for drugs in the solid-state, for drugs that are unstable in the stomach. Systems that prolong delivery ever the entire course of transit in the GI tract are beneficial. Compounds that are unstable in the small intestine may demonstrate decreased bioavailability when administered in the form of sustaining dosage form. This is because more drug is delivered in the small intestine and hence subject to degradation.

1.4.4 Plasma Half-Life

The usual goal of an oral sustained-release product is to maintain therapeutic blood levels over an extended period. To obtain such levels, a drug must enter in the circulation at approximately the same rate at which it is eliminated. The elimination rate is quantitatively described by the half-life ($t_{1/2}$). Therapeutic compounds with short half-lives are excellent candidates for sustained-release preparations. Since this can reduce dosing frequency. In general drugs with half-lives shorter than 2hrs are poor candidates of sustained release dosage whereas compounds with long half-lives, more than 6 hrs are also not used in sustained release forms because their effect is already sustained (Sahilhusen, et al., 2014; Garg, et al., 2013; Werle, et al., 2006; Varma, et al., 2004).

1.4.5 Therapeutic Window/ Index

The main goal for a formulation to be formulated as CR or modified release is to maintain the drug plasma level within an acceptable range of therapeutic window. This is a serious concern especially in the case of drugs having a shorter therapeutic index. Narrow therapeutic window drugs may face failure in such systems because of burst release.

1.5 References

Boyd, B. J., Whittaker, D. V., Khoo, S. M., & Davey, G. (2006). Lyotropic liquid crystalline phases formed from glycerate surfactants as sustained release drug delivery systems. *International journal of pharmaceutics, 309*(1-2), 218-226.

Colombo, P., Conte, U., Gazzaniga, A., Maggi, L., Sangalli, M. E., Peppas, N. A., & La Manna, A. (1990). Drug release modulation by physical restrictions of matrix swelling. *International journal of pharmaceutics, 63*(1), 43-48.

Gandhi, M., Chaudhari, R., Kulkarni, N., Bhusare, S., & Kare, P. (2014). Review article on pulsatile drug delivery system. *Int J Pharm Sci Rev Res, 26*, 251-255.

Garg, C., & Saluja, V. (2013). Once-daily sustained-release matrix tablets of metformin hydrochloride based on an enteric polymer and chitosan. *Journal of pharmaceutical education and research, 4*(1), 92.

Guru V. Betageri, Deepali V. Deshmukh and Ram B. Gupta, Oral sustained-release bioadhesive tablet formulation of didanosine, *Drug Development and Industrial Pharmacy*, 27 (2001): 129-136.

Herbert A. Lieberman, Leon Lachman and Joseph B. Schwartz, Pharmaceutical dosage forms, Tablets, Revised and Expanded 2(2003): 181.

Jain N.K. (2003), Advances in Controlled and Novel Drug Delivery. 1st edition, CBS Publishers & Distributors, New Dehli, India, 18. 293.

Jolly M. Sankalia, Mayur G. Sankalia, Rajashree C. Mashru, Drug release and swelling kinetics of directly compressed glipizide sustained-release matrices: Establishment of level A IVIVC. *Journal of Controlled Release*, 129 (2008): 49-58.

Kakar, S., Batra, D., & Singh, R. (2013). Preparation and evaluation of magnetic microspheres of mesalamine (5-aminosalicylic acid) for colon drug delivery. *Journal of acute disease*, 2(3), 226-231.

Prajapati, S. T., Patel, A. N., & Patel, C. N. (2011). Formulation and evaluation of controlled-release tablet of zolpidem tartrate by melt granulation technique. *International Scholarly Research Notices*, 2011.

Sahilhusen, I. J., Mukesh, R. P., & Alpesh, D. P. (2014). Sustained release drug delivery systems: a patent overview. *Aperito J Drug Designing and Pharmacology*, 1(1), 1-14.

Saikia, C., Gogoi, P., & Maji, T. K. (2015). Chitosan: A promising biopolymer in drug delivery applications. *J. Mol. Genet. Med. S*, 4(006), 899-910.

Sood, A., & Panchagnula, R. (2003). Design of controlled release delivery systems using a modified pharmacokinetic approach: a case study for drugs having a short elimination half-life and a narrow therapeutic index. *International journal of pharmaceutics*, 261(1-2), 27-41.

Varma, M. V., Kaushal, A. M., Garg, A., & Garg, S. (2004). Factors affecting mechanism and kinetics of drug release from matrix-based oral controlled drug delivery systems. *American Journal of drug delivery*, 2(1), 43-57

Wan, L. S., Heng, P. W., & Wong, L. F. (1993). Relationship between swelling and drug release in a hydrophilic matrix. *Drug development and industrial pharmacy*, 19(10), 1201-1210.

Muhammad Yasir Ali

Werle, M., & Bernkop-Schnürch, A. (2006). Strategies to improve plasma half life time of peptide and protein drugs. *Amino acids*, *30*(4), 351-367.

2. .POLYMERS

Saeed Ahmed

2.1. Introduction

Oral controlled drug delivery systems based on matrix type tablets are generally prepared by blending a drug and carrier material followed by compression. The carrier materials can be classified into water-insoluble carriers such as polymers (e.g. ethylcellulose, acrylate derivatives) or lipids (e.g. Gelucires) and water-soluble carriers. Water-soluble carriers (e.g. cellulose ethers, such as hydroxypropyl methylcellulose, polyoxyethylene oxide) have the advantage of complete erosion/dissolution and therefore no accumulation in the GI-tract as this is potentially possible with water-insoluble polymers (Sriwongjanya, et al., 1998).

Mundargi, et al., (2007) investigated the utilization of xanthan-grafted copolymer of acrylamide (AAM) in sustained-release (SR) matrix of Atenolol (ATL) and carvedilol (CDL). They used ATL and CDL as the active ingredient and microcrystalline cellulose (MCC), polyvinylpyrrolidone (K30), and Mg stearate, as excipients, in different concentrations.

Swellable matrix systems with anomalous release kinetics are suitable for drug release control for oral administration. The release rate modulation is achieved through the use of different types of polymer alone or in combinations. The drug release rate is linked to the properties and also the proportion of the drug the gel and the thickness of gel through which the drug must diffuse (Bodea, et al., 1997). Here are some of the polymers being used in matrix systems (Lachman, et al., 1991);

Table 2.1: Classification polymers based on solubility.

Polymer Types	Polymers
Insoluble, Inert	Polyethylene, PVC, EC
Insoluble, Erodidable	Carnuaba Wax, Stearic Acid, PEG, PEO
Hydrophilic	MC, HPMC, HEC
Polymer Types	**Polymers**
Natural	Alginates, Cellulose, Chitosan, Collagen, Polysaccharides,
Semisynthetic	Cellulose derivatives
Synthetic	Acrylic acid derivatives, PLGA, Polyamide, Polyether

2.2 Polymers

2.2.1 Hydroxypropyl Methylcellulose (HPMC)

Cellulose derivatives such as HPMC are used in hydrophilic matrix systems. It is one of the most commonly used hydrophilic vehicles used in the preparation of oral controlled drug delivery systems (Basak, et al. 2008). It is also known as Hypromellose, Hydroxypropyl methyl ether, etc. The chemical name is Cellulose, 2-hydroxypropyl methyl ether (Rowe, et al., 2009).

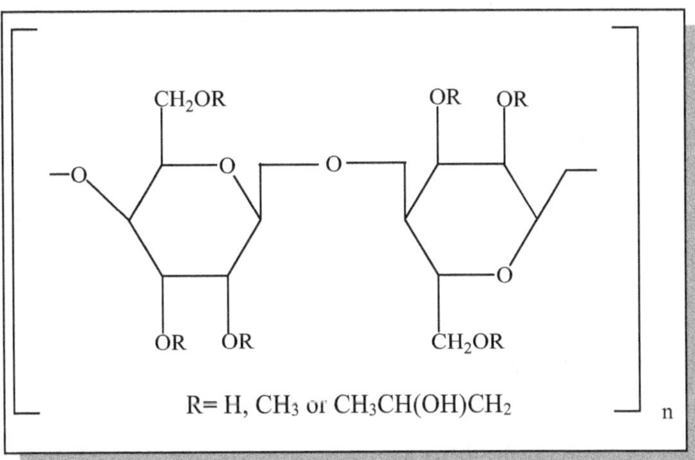

Figure 2.1: Structural formula of HPMC.

The substituent R in Figure represents either a methyl (–CH$_3$) or hydroxypropyl (-CH$_2$CHCH$_3$OH) or a hydrogen atom. The physicochemical properties of this polymer are strongly affected by;

a) Methoxyl group content
b) Hydroxypropyl group content
c) Molecular weight

HPMC is available in several grades that vary in viscosity and extent of substitution. The viscosity grade of the polymer depends on the number of substitutions on the polymeric backbone and the length of the cellulose chain. Two viscosity grades of HPMC (Methocel K100 and K4000) were extensively used as sustained release matrix polymers in the pharmaceutical industry. Among the various cellulose polymers used to prolong the drug release, HPMC has been widely used due to its rapid hydration, good compression and gelling characteristic, along with its ease of fabrication and very low toxicity (LD_{50} in the mouse: 5 g/kg) (Sung, et al., 1996).

Xu, et al. (2006) investigated the effect of formulations variables on the SR of Captopril. The excipients used were HPMC, microcrystalline cellulose (MCC), citric acid (CA), dibutyl phthalate, and PEG-400, and the dosage form was an elementary osmotic pump tablet. The core tablet was prepared using starch paste as a granulating agent. The granules were dried and then compressed. CA was used as the coating material. Then the effect of MCC and HPMC, present in the core tablet, was noted for CR. They found a good *in-vitro* and *in-vivo* correlation.

Srivastava, et al., (2005) studied floating matrix tablets developed for prolonged gastric residence time and to increase the bioavailability. He used the direct compression method for the preparation of matrix tablets. The amount of Atenolol (ATL) was 50 mg. Other ingredients were polymers HPMC (K15M, K4M), PVP (K30), sodium carboxymethylcellulose (SCMC), microcrystalline cellulose (MCC), guar gum (GG), and dicalcium phosphate (DCP). Besides these other chemicals were $NaHCO_3$, citric acid (CA), talc, and Mg-stearate. They found a prolonged release pattern of such systems in the presence of HPMC.

Gutierrez, et al., (2002) carried out a series of experiments for the test of the effect of different methocel grades (Methocel E, F, J, K) along with maltose, polyvinylpyrrolidone (PVP), PVA. Matrix tablets were used using Atenolol and PVP. Their extensive work on such formulations showed a sustained effect of polymers

Nur, et al., (2000) developed floating tablets of Captopril (CPTL). They use two grades of HPMC (4000 and 15000 cp) along with carbapol 934P. They mixed all the ingredients (excluding Mg-stearate and carbapol) and wet granulated with ethanol. After drying the granules at 40 °C overnight; the other two ingredients were added. They found that the hardness of tablets had a crucial effect on tablet buoyancy.

Iglesias, et al., (1998) worked on combined formulations of Atenolol (ATL) and Nifedipine (NFDN). They prepared ATL granules with lactose (using HPMC K100LV as the binder) and of that of NFDN by using different grades HPMC. Then both of these granules were mixed and tablets were compressed adding 0.5% w/w Mg-stearate as lubricating agent (drug to polymer ratio was 1:3). A sustained release pattern was obtained for ATL from these tablets.

2.2.2 Ethyl cellulose (EC)

EC is widely used in peroral sustained release dosage forms. It is synonymously known as Ethocel (Rowe, et al., 2009). It is an inert hydrophobic polymer and is essentially tasteless, odorless, and white tan-colored powder. It may be synthesis by the reaction of ethyl chloride with alkali cellulose, as shown below;

$$RONa + C_2H_5Cl \longrightarrow ROC_2H_5 + NaCl$$

Table 2.2: Different grades of HPMC and their viscosities.

Grades	Methoxyl (%)	Hydroxypropoxyl (%)	Viscosity of 2% soln. at 20°C (cP)
K100	19-24	7-12	80-120
K4M	19-24	7-12	3000–5600
K15M	19-24	7-12	11250–21000
K100M	19-24	7-12	80000–120000
E4M	28-30	7-12	3000–5600
E10M	28-30	7-12	7500–14000

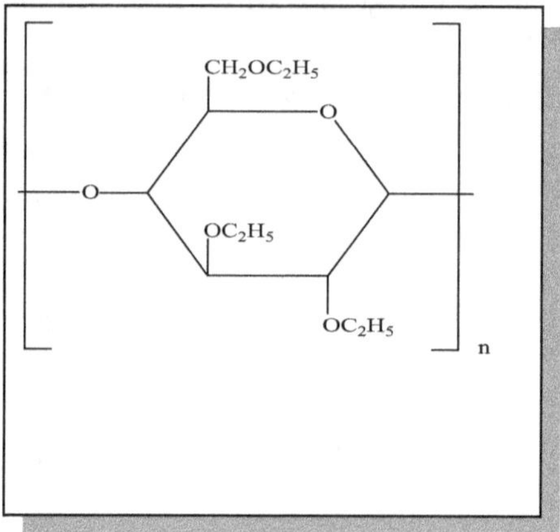

Figure 2.2: Structural formula of EC.

The main use of EC in oral formulations is as a hydrophobic coating agent for tablets and granules. EC coatings are used to modify the release of a drug, to mask the drug taste, and also to improve the stability of the tablets and granules from oxidation.

EC, for instance, does not erode or swell so modifies the release of the drug. Direct compression (Roy, et al., 2002) or wet granulation methods, using aqueous polymeric dispersion, (Muschert, et al., 2009; Khan, et al., 1998) both may be used for the preparation of tablets.

Stulzer, et al., (2008) formulated different CR CPTL formulations using methylcellulose (MC) and EC along with immediate-release tablets formulated using PVP. They formulated coated granules in a fluid bed dryer. They found that in the presence of EC/MC blend more than 12 hr release pattern was obtained as compared to tablets formulated in the presence of PVP.

Duarte, et al., (2006) prepared EC/MC microspheres by solvent system precipitation method, using dichloromethane (DCM) and dimethylsulfoxide (DMCO). The investigator checked the effect of different process variables on the CR effect of these blends precipitated. According to them, the best suitable conditions for successful formulations were 40 °C and 80 bar.

Samani, et al., (1999) evaluated the effects of different concentrations of various polysorbates on the release rate of ATL from film-coated tablets. Atenolol film-coated tablets were produced by mixing Atenolol, lactose, and PVP, granulating them with ethanol. Granules were dried and then tablets were coated with a 2 % solution of ethyl cellulose EC in dichloromethane. They found that the type of polymers had a less profound effect on the release kinetics of the drug.

Ho, et al., (1997) demonstrated the effect of granulated lactose or DCP with EC for CR of CPTL. They mixed lactose or DCP with HPMC and the mixture was then granulated with an aqueous solution of EC. The granules were then dried at 60 °C for 24 hr. 25 % w/w Captopril and 1% talc were initially blended with the granulated excipients prepared above. The mixture was then compressed to form tablets by direct compression. They demonstrated that the plasma concentrations of CPTL were less in the case of controlled-release preparations, showing a sustained effect of such preparations.

2.2.3 Hydroxyethyl Cellulose (HEC)

HEC occurs as a light tan or cream to white-colored, odorless, and tasteless hygroscopic powder. It is synonymously known as cellulose hydroxyethyl ether, ethyl hydroxy cellulose, etc (Rowe, et al., 2009).

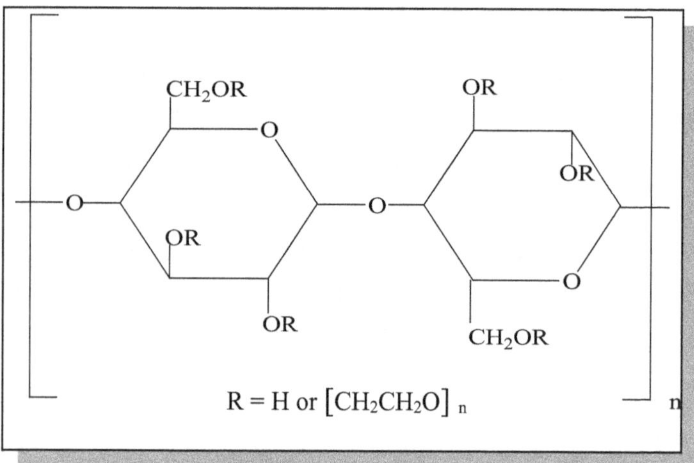

Figure 2.3: Structural formula of HEC.

It is a nonionic, water-soluble polymer widely used in pharmaceutical formulations. It is primarily used as a thickening agent in ophthalmic formulation along with binder and film coating agent in tablets. The nonionic polymers are very commonly used polymers in hydrophilic matrices because the rate of hydration of these polymers depends upon their degree of substitution. After the hydration, these form a gel around the formulation, just like HPMC, so the rate of drug release is controlled (Roy, et al., 2002).

2.2.4 Hydroxypropyl Cellulose (HPC)

It is white to slightly yellow-colored, odorless, and tasteless powder. Countless experiment results and theories have been published in the literature. HPC forms mesophases that can complicate solute transport due to the low hydrophilic nature as compared to the HPMC and HEC. An increasing trend of the hydrophilicity is shown as (Wise, 2000);

HPC ≈ MC < HPMC < HEC

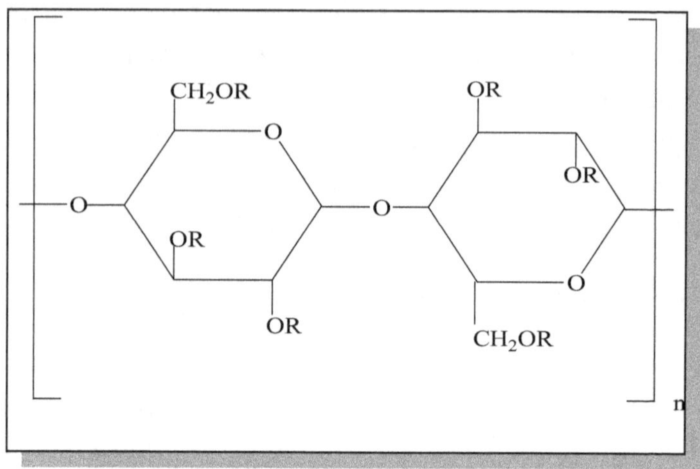

Figure 2.4: Structural formula of HPC.

The liquid penetration in HPC is less so there is less swelling as well as erosion as compared to others. HEC has 5-6 folds more swelling capacity as compared to that of HPC (Roy, et al., 2002). 15-35 % w/w of HPC may be used to produce sustained-release tablets. The sustained effect is decreased as the viscosity of HPC is decreased.

2.2.5 Chitosan (CS)

It occurs as an odorless, white or creamy-white powder or flakes, synonymously known as chitosan hydrochloride, chitosani hydrochloridum, 1-amino-2-deoxy-(1,4)-β-D-glucopyranose, etc (Rowe, et al., 2009).

$R = H \text{ or } [CH_2CHCH_2O]_n$

CS is repeating units of 1-amino-2-deoxy-(1,4)-β-D-glucopyranose but still small amount of 2-acetamido-2-deoxy-β-D-glucopyranose residues are also present. Grade having high amino acid content is water-soluble in aqueous acids. Three different forms are hydrated, dehydrated, and noncrystalline (Le, et al., 2003).

CS is a colon-specific drug delivery agent, may be used for the preparation of pH-based colon-specific drug delivery (Karanjit, et al. 2009). It may also be used in other dosage forms, e.g. gels, film (Chitosan) coated tables, microencapsulation, pellets, tablets, etc.

Rokhade, et al., (2007) formulated microspheres of theophylline with CS and MC blend. CS was dissolved in acetic acid solution and then MC was dispersed in this solution, theophylline was finally dissolved in the above-said dispersion. Liquid paraffin and glutaric acid were used for the microsphere preparation. They found the presence of drug profile extended for 12 hr. Moreover, the Fickian trend of release was observed.

Ikeda, et al., (2000) demonstrated the CR of CPTL using CS. They mixed the drug with different degrees of CS and a slurry was made by using water or ethanol (in one case water was used in the second ethanol was used as solvent). The slurry was dried and crushed to pass through 100 mesh size. This powder was filled in a hard gelatin capsule. They found a release profile of CPTL comparable to that of already marketed products.

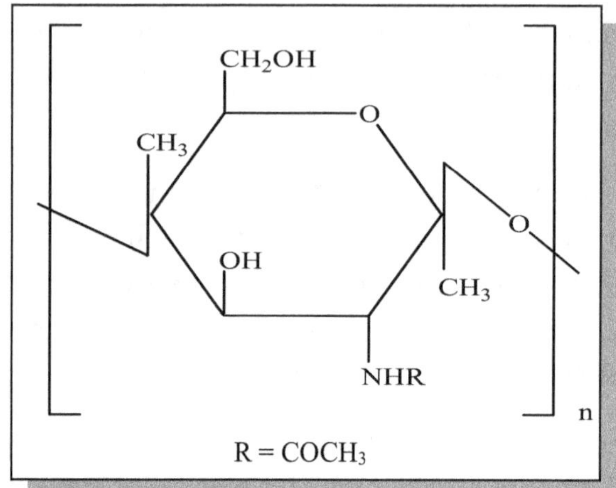

Figure 2.5: Structural formula of Chitosan.

2.2.6 Methylcellulose Glutarate (MCG)

Ali, et al., (2011) synthesized this novel polymeric system by reacting equimolar ration of MC with glutaric anhydride (esterification reaction). They used this for the preparation of CR matrix tablets of CPTL. They claim that tablets produced by this polymer showed zero-order release kinetics.

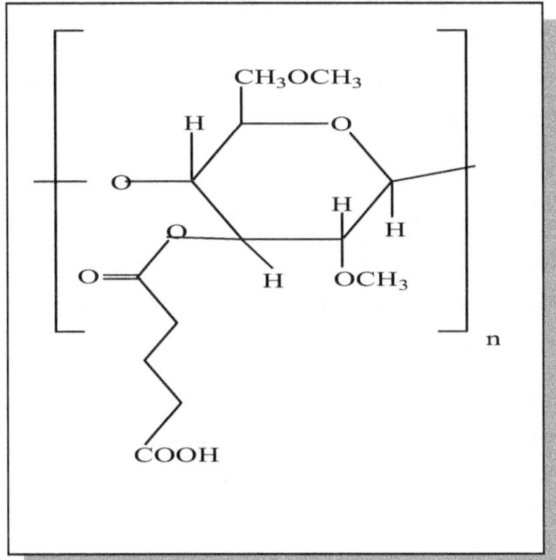

Figure 2.6: Structural formula of MCG.

2.3 References

Ali, Y., Ahmed, S., & Ahmed, I. (2011). Sustained release of captopril from matrix tablet using methylcellulose in a new derivative form. *Lat. Am. J. Pharm, 30*(9), 1696-1701.

Basak, S. C., Reddy, B. J., & Mani, K. L. (2006). Formulation and release behaviour of sustained release ambroxol hydrochloride HPMC matrix tablet. *Indian Journal of Pharmaceutical Sciences, 68*(5).

Bodea, A., & Leucuta, S. E. (1997). Optimization of hydrophilic matrix tablets using a D-optimal design. *International journal of pharmaceutics, 153*(2), 247-255.

Duarte, A. R. C., Gordillo, M. D., Cardoso, M. M., Simplício, A. L., & Duarte, C. M. (2006). Preparation of ethyl cellulose/methyl cellulose blends by supercritical antisolvent precipitation. *International journal of pharmaceutics*, *311*(1-2), 50-54.

Gutierrez-Rocca, J., & Dunne, J. (2002). *U.S. Patent No. 6,491,950*. Washington, DC: U.S. Patent and Trademark Office.

Ho, H. O., Wang, H. Y., & Sheu, M. T. (1997). The evaluation of granulated excipients as matrix material for controlled delivery of captopril. *Journal of controlled release*, *49*(2-3), 243-251.

Iglesias, R., Taboada, C., Souto, C., Martinez-Pacheco, R., Gomez-Amoza, J. L., & Concheiro, A. (1998). Development of tablets for controlled joint release of nifedipine and atenolol. *Drug development and industrial pharmacy*, *24*(9), 835-840.

Ikeda, Y., Kimura, K., Hirayama, F., Arima, H., & Uekama, K. (2000). Controlled release of a water-soluble drug, captopril, by a combination of hydrophilic and hydrophobic cyclodextrin derivatives. *Journal of controlled release*, *66*(2-3), 271-280.

Khan, G. M., & Zhu, J. B. (1998). Ibuprofen release kinetics from controlled-release tablets granulated with aqueous polymeric dispersion of ethylcellulose II: Influence of several parameters and coexcipients. *Journal of controlled release*, *56*(1-3), 127-134.

Lachman, L., Lieberman, H. A., & Kanig, J. L. (1991). "Granulation", The Theory and practice of industrial pharmacy.

Le Tien, C., Lacroix, M., Ispas-Szabo, P., & Mateescu, M. A. (2003). N-acylated chitosan: hydrophobic matrices for controlled drug release. *Journal of Controlled Release*, *93*(1), 1-13.

Mundargi, R. C., Patil, S. A., & Aminabhavi, T. M. (2007). Evaluation of acrylamide-grafted-xanthan gum copolymer matrix tablets for oral controlled delivery of antihypertensive drugs. *Carbohydrate Polymers*, *69*(1), 130-141.

Muschert, S., Siepmann, F., Leclercq, B., Carlin, B., & Siepmann, J. (2009). Drug release mechanisms from ethylcellulose: PVA-PEG graft copolymer-coated pellets. *European Journal of Pharmaceutics and Biopharmaceutics*, *72*(1), 130-137.

Nur, A. O., & Zhang, J. S. (2000). Captopril floating and/or bioadhesive tablets: design and release kinetics. *Drug development and industrial pharmacy*, *26*(9), 965-969.

Rokhade, A. P., Shelke, N. B., Patil, S. A., & Aminabhavi, T. M. (2007). Novel interpenetrating polymer network microspheres of chitosan and methylcellulose for controlled release of theophylline. *Carbohydrate Polymers*, *69*(4), 678-687.

Rowe, R. C., Sheskey, P., & Quinn, M. (2009). *Handbook of pharmaceutical excipients*. Libros Digitales-Pharmaceutical Press.

Roy, D. S., & Rohera, B. D. (2002). Comparative evaluation of rate of hydration and matrix erosion of HEC and HPC and study of drug release from their matrices. *European Journal of Pharmaceutical Sciences*, *16*(3), 193-199.

Samani, S. M., Adrangui, M., Farid, D. J., & Nokhodchi, A. (1999). Effect of polysorbates on atenolol release from film-coated tablets. *Drug development and industrial pharmacy*, *25*(4), 513-516.

Srivastava, A. K., Wadhwa, S., Ridhurkar, D., & Mishra, B. (2005). Oral sustained delivery of atenolol from floating matrix tablets—formulation and *in vitro* evaluation. *Drug development and industrial pharmacy*, *31*(4-5), 367-374.

Sriwongjanya, M., & Bodmeier, R. (1998). Effect of ion exchange resins on the drug release from matrix tablets. *European journal of pharmaceutics and biopharmaceutics, 46*(3), 321-327.

Stulzer, H. K., Segatto Silva, M. A., Fernandes, D., & Assreuy, J. (2008). Development of controlled release captopril granules coated with ethylcellulose and methylcellulose by fluid bed dryer. *Drug delivery, 15*(1), 11-18.

Sung, K. C., Nixon, P. R., Skoug, J. W., Ju, T. R., Gao, P., Topp, E. M., & Patel, M. V. (1996). Effect of formulation variables on drug and polymer release from HPMC-based matrix tablets. *International journal of pharmaceutics, 142*(1), 53-60.

Wise, D. L. (2000). *Handbook of pharmaceutical controlled release technology.* CRC press.

Xu, L., Li, S., & Sunada, H. (2006). Preparation and evaluation in vitro and in vivo of captopril elementary osmotic pump tablets. *Asian J Pharm Sci, 1*(3-4), 236-245.

3. OSMOTIC SYSTEMS

Muhammad Yasir Ali
Ghulam Abbas

3.1 Introduction

Osmotic drug delivery technology is primarily based on the semipermeable membrane. These membranes are permeable only to water but not permeable to ionic or high molecular weight compounds. They are also known as the gastrointestinal therapeutic system (Syed, et al., 2015; Keraliya, et al., 2012).

3.1.1 Advantage

Osmotic pumps have the following advantages over conventional dosage forms (Sharma, et al., 2018; Patel, et al., 2017);

a) Osmotic systems usually give a zero-order drug release pattern.

b) Drug release is free of environmental variables at the site of drug release.

c) The release mechanisms are independent of the nature of the drug.

d) A good level of *in-vitro* and *in-vivo* correlation is present.

e) Decreased level of side effects is present due to predefined factors.

f) Patient compliance is high due to decrease drug frequency.

3.1.2 Disadvantage

As multiple excipients and steps are required for the preparation of such critical systems, hence, there are some disadvantages of osmotic pumps, as follows (Sharma, et al., 2018; Patel, et al., 2017);

a) Extensive work is required to prepare so these are costly.

b) Dose dumping may be present if the coating process is not well controlled or defective.

c) The delivery hole and its size are critical.

d) It may cause irritation due to the release of a saturated solution of the drug.

3.2 Historic Back Ground

3.2.1 Rose-Nelson Pump

Two Australian physiologists Rose and Nelson, in 1955, developed a system. They developed a system in which water and salt compartments are separated by a semi-permeable membrane (Figure 3.1). On the other hand, the salt and drug compartment are separated by an elastic diaphragm. The difference in osmotic pressure across the membrane moves water from the water compartment into a salt compartment. Due to the osmotic pull and movement of water, the salt compartment will expand. This expansion creates pressure on the diaphragm present between the salt and drug compartment. This results in the release of the drug (Keraliya, et al., 2012; Gosh, et al., 2011; Rose, et al., 1955).

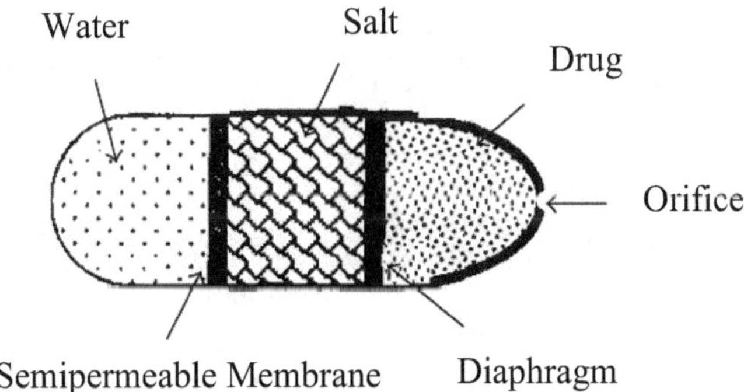

Figure 3.1: Rose-Nelson pump.

3.2.2 Higuchi-Leeper Pump

A variation in the Rose Nelson pump is present in the form of the Higuchi Leeper Pump as shown in Figure 3.2. This is a simplified version of a previously prepared osmotic pump and has differences only in the absence of a water chamber. The rest of the principle is the same, except, it takes water from the surrounding environment. The moveable separator or diaphragm pushes drug content out through the orifice after the osmotic pressure is built inside the device due to the presence of $MgSO_4$. In this, the pump can be prepared and stored for an extended period before it is used (Singh, et al., 2013; Keraliya, et al., 2012).

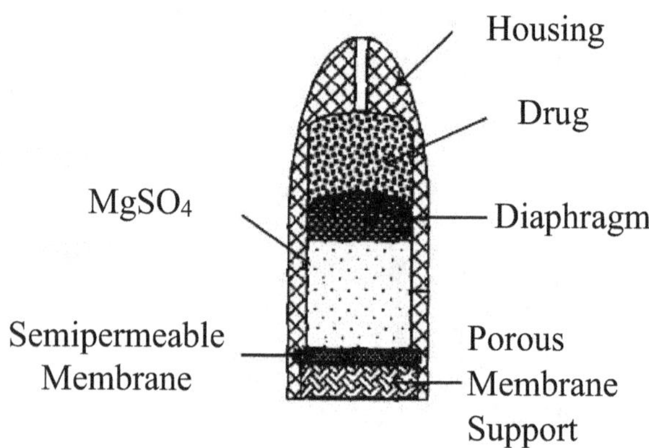

Figure 3.2: Higuchi-Leeper pump.

3.2.3 Higuchi-Theeuwes Pump

Another modification in the Rose Nelson pump was the development of a new device in which a semipermeable membrane acts as outer support or housing, itself. This system also lacks a water compartment. However, upon exposure to the aqueous medium, osmotic pressure is developed and the salt chamber thus pushes the drug to release from these devices through the orifice (Mathur, et al., 2016; Singh, et al., 2013; Keraliya, et al., 2012).

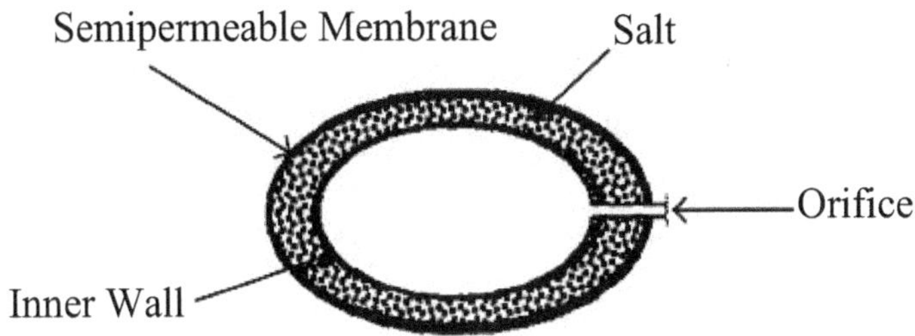

Figure 3.3: Higuchi-Theeuwes pump.

3.3 Types of Osmotic Pumps

Depending upon their fabrication and the variations in the active ingredient, osmotic devices can be classified as follows:

3.3.1 Elementary-Osmotic Pump (EOP)

This pump is an excellent example of a dosage form that has limited or no effect of GIT factors such as pH or motility. The dosage form is made by blending of drug and suitable osmogene. The blend is covered with some semipermeable membrane, acting both as rate controlling membrane and as well as a coating material. A hole is drilled through the layer in the coating material. After coming in contact with the aqueous medium, water goes inside the device through this hole and a concentrated solution is obtained. Then the drug content is released from the same orifice. The demerits of the EOP are that these systems are suitable only for the delivery of water-soluble drugs (Sharma, et al., 2018; Gupt, et al., 2010).

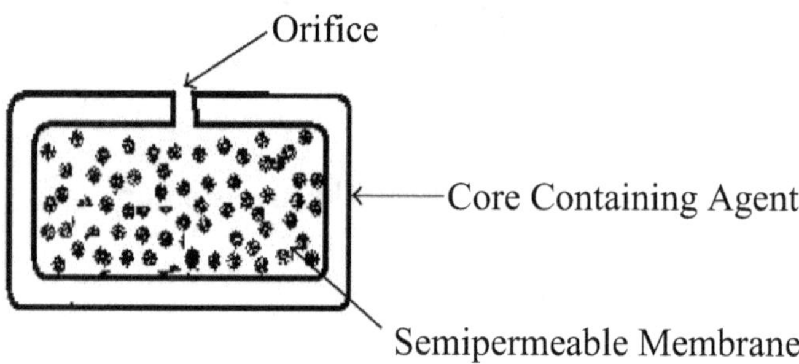

Figure 3.4: Elementary-Osmotic pump.

3.3.2 Push-Pull Osmotic Pump (PPOP)

The push-pull osmotic pump is a typical example of modification of EOP. This system was developed to load both water-soluble and water-insoluble both kinds of drug. Thus, PPOP overcomes the problem of non-suitability of water-insoluble drugs as in the case of EOP. The PPOP contains two layers (Figure 3.5). The upper layer is composed of drugs and some required excipients. On the other hand, the second layer contains osmogene and remaining excipients. This two-core system is covered with a semipermeable membrane. A hole is drilled through this membrane on the side of the drug core. When PPOP comes in contact with water, the layer containing osmogene swells, creating pressure on the drug layer. This results in the release of the drug through the orifice in the form of solution or suspension (Zhao, et al., 2015; Wu, et al., 2014; Keraliya, et al., 2012).

3.3.3 Sandwiched Osmotic Tablet (SOT)

Sandwiched osmotic tablets represent another modification of old systems. This device is composed of a central compartment of osmogene. The osmogene is covered with the drug-excipient mixture from two sides. The semipermeable membrane acts as the outer layer of the systems. Two holes are drilled with a coating front near the drug compartment. When SOT comes in contact with GIT fluids, the push layer containing the osmogenes swells, and the drug is released from the two release orifices present on the sides of the tablet (Shirole, et al., 2020; Gupta, et al., 2010).

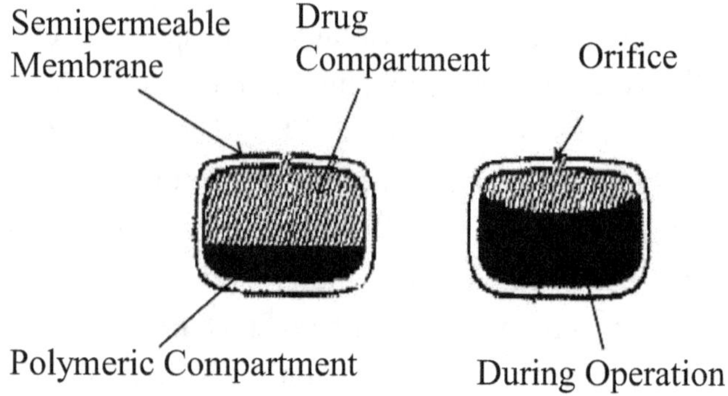

Figure 3.5: Push-Pull pump.

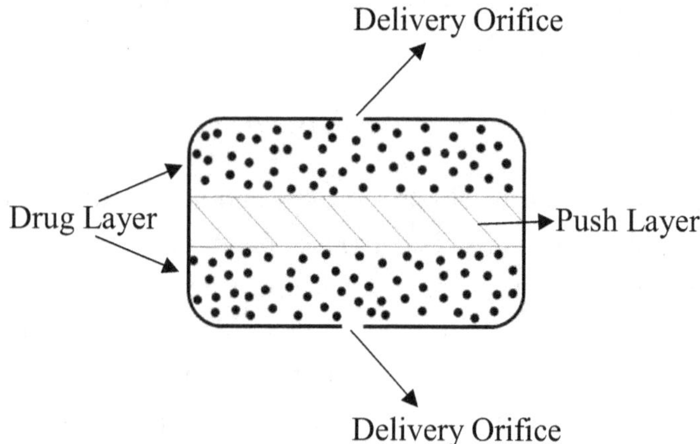

Figure 3.6: Sandwiched-Osmotic tablet (SOT).

3.4 Factors Affecting the Release Rate

The following factors should be kept in mind while designing an osmotic pump.

3.4.1 Type of Membrane

The release of drugs from osmotic devices is independent of the pH and other environmental factors such as the site of release. The presence of a water-only permeable membrane and separation of dissolution of drug core from GIT environment. The membrane in the osmotic system is semi-permeable in nature. All the polymers permeable to water but impermeable to active agents and excipients can be used. The examples include cellulose ethers and esters e.g. ethylcellulose and Eudragit. Among the cellulose polymer, cellulose acetate membranes are mostly used because of their high water permeability characteristics and they can be accustomed to a different degree of acetylation. The permeability of this membrane can be amplified by adding a plasticizer to the polymer if required.

3.4.2 Membrane Thickness

One of the main factors influencing the rate of water penetration into the core of osmotic pumps is the thickness of the semipermeable membrane. The water permeability into the membrane can be enhanced by the choice of a suitable type of membrane material. However, the release rate can be controlled by making some changes to the membrane materials. A single agent, as well as a good mixture of different polymers, can be used to make the release rate of your own choice.

3.4.3 Osmotic Pressure

Osmogenes uphold a concentration gradient across the membrane. They also enhance the uptake of water and thus help to make uniformly hydrated formulations. The rate of water flow can be calculated as follows;

$$d_V/d_t = A\ \theta\ \Delta\pi/l$$

d_V/d_t = flow of water

A = membrane area

Θ = permeability

$\Delta\pi$ = difference of osmotic gradient of two different solution fronts

L = membrane thickness

3.4.4 Osmotic Agents
Inorganic water-soluble osmogenes

a) KCl

b) $MgSO_4$

c) NaCl

d) $NaHCO_3$

e) $NaSO_4$

Organic polymer osmogenes

a) Citric acid

b) Fructose

c) Fructose/Dextrose

d) Fructose/Lactose

c) Lactose

f) Mannitol

g) Sorbitol

h) Sucrose

i)   Sucrose/Fructose

j)   Sucrose/Lactose

3.4.5 Plasticizers

The presence of plasticizers may also play its role in the rate-controlling mechanism of drug release. The chemical nature of plasticizers and their concentrations are factors influencing these formulations. The key participation of such materials is to change the elastic behavior of the membrane which then can modify the release pattern after changing the permeability of the membrane. A few examples are as follow (Sahoo, et al., 2015; Verma, et al., 2002);

a)   Alkyl adipates

b)   Benzoates

c)   Glycolates

d)   Glycolates

e)   Myristates

f)   Myristates

g)   Phathalates

h)   Phenyls

i) Propionates

j) Sulphonamides

3.4.6 Delivery Orifice

Amongst all others, the orifice is one of the crucial components of coating membrane for the release of the drug. The critical control over the size of the orifice is a pre-requisite of the successful osmotic pump. The use of laser or indentation in the membrane at the site may be used for the creation of orifice/orifices in the membrane.

3.4.7 Solubility

Solubility parameters of the drug in the case of the EOP may be one of the utmost significant factors factor affecting the drug release kinetics. The amount of drugs from such systems with zero-order release patterns can be calculated as the equation given below. The drug with the solubility of ≤ 0.05 g/cm^2 would release the drug $\geq 95\ \%$ by the zero-order kinetics according to the equation.

$$F_{(z)} = 1-S/\rho$$

$F_{(z)}$ = fraction of drug released

S = drug solubility

ρ = core density

3.4.8 Wicking Agents

These agents help in enhancing the surface area of the drug in contact with the environment. Their presence increases the release rate of the drug through the delivery orifice. Alumina, bentonite, collodion, niacinamide, polyester, polyvinyl pyrrolidone, silicon dioxide, and sodium lauryl sulfate are a few examples of wicking agents used in osmotic pumps.

3.4.9 Coating Solvents

Nearly all kinds of sole solvent (inorganic or organic) or a mixture of solvents can be used for the coating of core osmotic systems. The typical solvents include alcohols, acetone, cyclohexane, and water, etc. Co-solvency of acetone/methanol, acetone/ethanol, acetone/water, methylene chloride/methanol etc. can be used.

3.5 References

Ghosh, T., & Ghosh, A. (2011). Drug delivery through osmotic systems—an overview. *Journal of Applied Pharmaceutical Science, 2*, 38-49.

Gupta, B. P., Thakur, N., Jain, N. P., Banweer, J., & Jain, S. (2010). Osmotically controlled drug delivery system with associated drugs. *Journal of Pharmacy & Pharmaceutical Sciences, 13*(4), 571-588.

Keraliya, R. A., Patel, C., Patel, P., Keraliya, V., Soni, T. G., Patel, R. C., &z Patel, M. M. (2012). Osmotic drug delivery system as a part of modified release dosage form. *International Scholarly Research Notices*, *2012*.

Mathur, M., & Mishra, R. (2016). A review on osmotic pump drug delivery system. *International journal of pharmaceutical sciences and research*, *7*(2), 453.

Patel, H. J., & Parikh, V. P. (2017). An overview of osmotic drug delivery system: an update review. *Int J Bioassays*, *6*(7), 5426-36.

Rose, S., & Nelson, J. F. (1955). A continuous long-term injector. *Australian Journal of Experimental Biology and Medical Science*, *33*(4), 415-420.

Sahoo, C. K., Sahoo, N. K., Rao, S. R. M., Sudhakar, M., & Satyanarayana, K. (2015). A review on controlled porosity osmotic pump tablets and its evaluation. *Bulletin of Faculty of Pharmacy, Cairo University*, *53*(2), 195-205.

Sharma, A., Kumar, D., & Painuly, N. (2018). A review on osmotically controlled drug delivery systems. *Asian Journal of Pharmaceutical Research and Development*, *6*(4), 101-109.

Shirole, P. U., Patil, P. B., & Bachhav, R. S. (2020). Review on osmotic drug delivery system. *IJRAR-International Journal of Research and Analytical Reviews (IJRAR)*, *7*(2), 7-22.

Singh, K., Walia, M. K., Agarwal, G., & Harikumar, S. L. (2013). Osmotic pump drug delivery system: a noval approach. *Journal of Drug Delivery and Therapeutics*, *3*(5), 156-162.

Syed, S. M. (2015). Osmotic Drug Delivery System: An Overview. *International journal of Pharmaceutical research & Allied sciences*, *4*(3).

Verma, R. K., Krishna, D. M., & Garg, S. (2002). Formulation aspects in the development of osmotically controlled oral drug delivery systems. *Journal of controlled release, 79*(1-3), 7-27.

Wu, C., Zhao, Z., Zhao, Y., Hao, Y., Liu, Y., & Liu, C. (2014). Preparation of a push–pull osmotic pump of felodipine solubilized by mesoporous silica nanoparticles with a core–shell structure. *International journal of pharmaceutics, 475*(1-2), 298-305.

Zhao, Z., Wu, C., Zhao, Y., Hao, Y., Liu, Y., & Zhao, W. (2015). Development of an oral push–pull osmotic pump of fenofibrate-loaded mesoporous silica nanoparticles. *International journal of nanomedicine, 10,* 1691.

4. MATRIX SYSTEMS

Nisar-ur-Rahman

4.1 Matrix Controlled Release Systems

A matrix device is a drug delivery system in which the drug is dispersed either molecularly or in a particulate form within a polymeric network. The device may be a swellable, hydrophilic monolithic system, an erosion-controlled monolithic system, or a non-erodible system (Roy, et al., 2002; Cardinal, 1984).

4.2 TYPES OF MATRICES

Matrix system tablets are the most common device for controlling the release of drugs. This is possible because they are relatively easy to fabricate as compared to membrane/ barrier controlled systems and less chance of accidental toxic dose to occur, which could be the result of rupturing of membrane or barrier in membrane controlled systems. There are two systems present in this class of dosage form;

Hydrophilic matrix systems

Hydrophobic matrix systems

Both hydrophilic and hydrophobic matrix systems are widely used to provide controlled (sustained) delivery of drug substances because of their versatility, effectiveness, and low cost. These types of systems are also suitable for in-house development since they are usually manufactured using conventional types of equipment and processing. In a matrix system, a drug is incorporated into the polymer matrix by either particle or molecular dispersion. The former is simply a suspension of drug particles homogeneously distributed in the polymer matrix, whereas the latter is a matrix with drug molecules dissolved in the polymer (Wise, 2005).

4.2.1 Hydrophilic Matrix Systems (Hydrogels)

Hydrogels are three-dimensional, water-swollen structures composed of mainly hydrophilic homopolymers or copolymers. They are rendered insoluble due to cross-link b chemical bonds, or other cohesion forces such as ionic interaction, hydrogen bonding, or hydrophobic interaction. Hydrogels are elastic solids in the sense that there exists a remembered reference configuration to which the system returns even after being deformed for a very long time (Jain, 2004).

In recent years, considerable attention has been focused on hydrophilic polymers in the design of oral controlled drug delivery systems because of their flexibility to obtain a desirable drug release profile, cost-effectiveness, and broad regulatory acceptance (Al-Saidan, et al., 2005).

Cumulative evidence suggests that hydrogels pose such unique properties that make them a highly acceptable and sophisticated systems for controlled drug delivery (Jain, 2008).

a) They are highly biocompatible.

b) They have low interfacial tension with surrounding biological fluid and tissues, which minimizes the driving force for protein adsorption and cell adhesion.

c) Low friction surfaces cause no pain and damage to mucous membranes or the intima of the blood vessels due to soft rubbery nature and thus no infection thrombus formation.

d) The release of the therapeutic agent can be regulated by controlling swelling and cross-linking density.

e) It can be supplied for both hydrophilic and hydrophobic drugs and charged solutes.

f) Relatively easy extraction of polymerization initiators, decomposition products, and polymerization solvents prior to in vivo application.

g) Hydrogels simulate some hydrodynamic properties of natural biological gels, cells, and tissues.

Commonly available hydrophilic polymers include hydroxypropyl methylcellulose (HPMC), hydroxypropyl cellulose (HPC), hydroxyethylcellulose (HEC), xanthan gum, sodium alginate, poly(ethylene oxide), and cross-linked homopolymers, and copolymers of acrylic acid. They are mostly supplied in micronized forms because the small particle size is critical to the rapid formation of the gelatinous layer on the tablet surface.

4.2.2 Hydrophobic Matrix Systems

Hydrophobic and monolithic polymer matrix systems usually use waxes and water-insoluble polymers in their formulation. Many waxes are long carbon chain wax esters, glycerides, and fatty acids. Natural and synthetic waxes of differing melting points have been used as controlled release matrix materials (Wise, 2005).

There are different types of polymers used for this sort of dosage form to be developed along with the above-mentioned polymers. These are ethyl cellulose (Ethocel FP7, FP 10, FP100), acrylate derivatives (Eudragit RL100, PO, RS100, PO), cellulose acetate (CA-398-10), cellulose acetate butyrate (CAB-381-20), cellulose acetate propionate (CAB-482-20) (Wise, 2005; Sriwongjanya, et al., 1998).

4.3 Matrix System Production Method

There are many different methods for the production of matrix tablets. These are given below;

Wet granulation

Direct compression

4.4 *In Vitro* Evaluation of Tablets

4.4.1 Experimental Conditions

The *in vitro* analysis of tablet is done by the following test (see section 7.6);

a) Weight variation test
b) Hardness testing
c) Friability
d) Dissolution

4.4.2 Assessment of Matrices

Drug release profiles can be evaluated by different kinetic models (Ali, et al., 2011; Bravo, et al., 2004; Tahara, et al., 1995). In addition, the similarity factor is also sometimes checked to compare the formulations (Aslam, et al., 2012; Farago, et al., 2008).

Table 4.1: Conditions recommended for dissolution testing of controlled release dosage forms.

Media	1. Water
	2. Buffer of pH 1-1.5, 4-4.5, 6-7.4
	3. Simulated gastric fluid
Mixing	50 rpm, 100 rpm, 150 rpm
Sampling time	0, 0.5, 01, 1.5, 02, 03, 04, 06, 08, 10, 12 hr
Temperature	$37.5 \pm 0.5\ ^{\circ}C$

4.4.2.1 Model Dependent Approaches

Zero-order equation: $Q = k_0\, t$

Where Q is the amount of drug released at time t and k_0 is the release rate constant (Khan, et al., 2010). The graph for the zero-order kinetic model is plotted between the cumulative amount of drug released versus time. This relationship can be used to describe the drug dissolution of several types of modified release pharmaceutical dosage forms, as in the case of some matrices, transdermal systems, as well as matrix tablets with low soluble drugs in coated forms, osmotic systems, etc. In most of the cases, the rate-limiting ingredient is the polymer used to fabricate the matrix.

First-order equation: $\ln[(C_\infty - C_t)/C_\infty] = -kt$

Where C_0 is the initial concentration of the drug, k is the first-order rate constant, and t is the time (Butterworth, et al., 2012; Khan, et al., 2010). The data obtained are plotted as log cumulative percentage of drug remaining versus time which would yield a straight line with a slope of -K/2.303. This relationship can be used to describe the drug dissolution in pharmaceutical dosage forms such as those containing water-soluble drugs in porous matrices.

Higuchi square root equation: $Q = k_H \, t^{0.5}$

Where k_H is the Higuchi rate constant.

According to this model, the initial drug concentration is relatively higher, which results in the bulk release of the drug from outer surfaces and layers of the matrix system. After some time, the drug starts to release from channels or pores created in the matrix bed. This results in constant drug diffusion from the matrix core. The data obtained were plotted as cumulative percentage drug release versus square root of time (Shah, et al., 2012; Paul, et al., 2011; Higuchi, et al., 1963).

This relationship can be used to describe the drug dissolution from several types of modified release pharmaceutical dosage forms, as in the case of some transdermal systems and matrix tablets with water-soluble drugs.

Hixson-Crowell model: $W_0^{1/3} - W_t^{1/3} = \kappa \, t$

Where W_0 is the initial amount of drug in the pharmaceutical dosage form, Wt is the remaining amount of drug in the pharmaceutical dosage form at time t and κ is a constant incorporating the surface-volume relation (Craciun, et al., 2019; Panotopoulos, et al., 2019). The equation describes the release from systems where there is a change in surface area and diameter of particles or tablets. To study the release kinetics, data obtained from *in vitro* drug release studies were plotted as the cube root of drug percentage remaining in matrix *versus* time.

This expression applies to pharmaceutical dosage forms such as tablets, where the dissolution occurs in planes that are parallel to the drug surface if the tablet dimensions diminish proportionally, in such a manner that the initial geometrical form keeps constant all the time (Craciun, et al., 2019).

Korsmeyer-Peppas model: $M_t / M_\infty = kt^n$

Where M_t / M_∞ is the fractional drug release at time t, k is kinetic constant and n is the so-called diffusion exponent, indicative of the mechanism of the drug release. The equation generally holds for $M_t/M_\infty > 70\%$ of drug release. $N = 0.45$ or $0.45 < n < 0.89$ or $n > 0.89$, indicates Fickian diffusion or anomalous transport or Case ''II'' transport kinetics respectively (Wu, et al., 2019; Peppas, et al., 1997).

4.4.2.2 Model Independent Approaches

FDA suggests a model-independent approach for the comparison of two formulations at a particular time. This method relies on the calculation of drug release at a specific time and then putting the values in the equation. Rt and Tt are the percent drug released at a given time point. similarity factor (f_2) having a value between 50 and 100 indicate equivalence in dissolution profiles. If $f_2 = 100$. This means that the dissolution profiles for the reference and test products overlap and are identical (Aslam, et al., 2012; Soni, et al., 2008).

$$f_2 = 50 \bullet \log \left\{ \left[1 + \left(\frac{1}{n} \sum (R_t - T_t)^2 \right]^{-0.5} \bullet 100 \right. \right\}$$

4.5 Reference

Ali, Y., Ahmed, S., & Ahmed, I. (2011). Sustained release of captopril from matrix tablet using methylcellulose in a new derivative form. *Lat. Am. J. Pharm*, *30*(9), 1696-1701.

Al-Saidan, S. M., Krishnaiah, Y. S., Patro, S., & Satyanaryana, V. (2005). *In vitro* and in vivo evaluation of guar gum matrix tablets for oral controlled release of water-soluble diltiazem hydrochloride. *Aaps Pharmscitech*, *6*(1), E14-E21.

Aslam, Z., Akhter, K. P., Ahmad, M., Aamir, M. N., Naeem, M., & Ali, M. Y. (2012). Preparation of modified-release tramadol tablets and drug release evaluation using dependent and independent modeling approaches. *Lat. Am. J. Pharm*, *31*(10), 1417-21.

Bravo, S. A., Lamas, M. C., & Salomon, C. J. (2004). Swellable matrices for the controlled-release of diclofenac sodium: Formulation and in vitro studies. *Pharmaceutical development and technology*, *9*(1), 75-83.

Butterworth, P. J., Warren, F. J., Grassby, T., Patel, H., & Ellis, P. R. (2012). Analysis of starch amylolysis using plots for first-order kinetics. *Carbohydrate Polymers*, *87*(3), 2189-2197.

Cardinal, J. R. (1984). Drug release from matrix devices. In *Recent advances in drug delivery systems* (pp. 229-248). Springer, Boston, MA.

Craciun, A. M., Barhalescu, M. L., Agop, M., & Ochiuz, L. (2019). Theoretical modeling of long-time drug release from nitrosalicyl-imine-chitosan hydrogels through multifractal logistic type laws. *Computational and mathematical methods in medicine*, *2019*.

Farago, P. V., Raffin, R. P., Pohlmann, A. R., Guterres, S. S., & Zawadzki, S. F. (2008). Physicochemical characterization of a hydrophilic model drug-loaded PHBV microparticles obtained by the double emulsion/solvent evaporation technique. *Journal of the Brazilian Chemical Society*, *19*(7), 1298-1305.

Higuchi, T. (1963). Mechanism of sustained-action medication. Theoretical analysis of rate of release of solid drugs dispersed in solid matrices. *Journal of pharmaceutical sciences*, *52*(12), 1145-1149.

Jain, N. K. (Ed.). (2008). *Advances in controlled and novel drug delivery*. CBS Publishers & Distributors.

Khan, S. A., Ahmad, M., Aamir, M. N., Murtaza, G., Rasool, F., & Akhtar, M. (2010). Study of nimesulide release from ethylcellulose microparticles and drug-polymer compatibility analysis. *Lat. Am. J. Pharm*, *29*(4), 554-561.

Panotopoulos, G. P., & Haidar, Z. S. (2019). Mathematical Modeling for Pharmaco-Kinetic and-Dynamic Predictions from Controlled Drug Release NanoSystems: A Comparative Parametric Study. *Scientifica, 2019*.

Paul, D. R. (2011). Elaborations on the Higuchi model for drug delivery. *International journal of pharmaceutics*, *418*(1), 13-17.

Peppas, N. A., & Colombo, P. (1997). Analysis of drug release behavior from swellable polymer carriers using the dimensionality index. *Journal of Controlled Release*, *45*(1), 35-40.

Roy, D. S., & Rohera, B. D. (2002). Comparative evaluation of rate of hydration and matrix erosion of HEC and HPC and study of drug release from their matrices. *European Journal of Pharmaceutical Sciences*, *16*(3), 193-199.

Shah, K. U., & Khan, G. M. (2012). Regulating drug release behavior and kinetics from matrix tablets based on fine particle-sized ethyl cellulose ether derivatives: an in vitro and in vivo evaluation. *The Scientific World Journal, 2012*.

Soni, T. G., Desai, J. U., Nagda, C. D., Gandhi, T. R., & Chotai, N. P. (2008). Mathematical evaluation of similarity factor using various weighing approaches on aceclofenac marketed formulations by model-independent method. *Die Pharmazie-An International Journal of Pharmaceutical Sciences*, *63*(1), 31-34.

Sriwongjanya, M., & Bodmeier, R. (1998). Effect of ion exchange resins on the drug release from matrix tablets. *European journal of pharmaceutics and biopharmaceutics*, *46*(3), 321-327.

Tahara, K., Yamamoto, K., & Nishihata, T. (1995). Overall mechanism behind matrix sustained release (SR) tablets prepared with hydroxypropyl methylcellulose 2910. *Journal of controlled release, 35*(1), 59-66.

Wise, D. L. (2000). *Handbook of pharmaceutical controlled release technology.* CRC press.

Wu, I. Y., Bala, S., Škalko-Basnet, N., & Di Cagno, M. P. (2019). Interpreting non-linear drug diffusion data: Utilizing Korsmeyer-Peppas model to study drug release from liposomes. *European Journal of Pharmaceutical Sciences, 138*, 105026.

5. FLOATING DRUG DELIVERY SYSTEMS

Romna Tul Janat

5.1 Introduction

Gastric emptying of dosage forms is an immensely changeable process and the capacity to enhance and control the emptying time is an important forte for dosage forms, which, as compared to the conventional dosage forms, resides in the stomach for a prolonged period (Whitehead, et al., 1998). Various problems are faced while designing controlled release systems for greater absorption and improved bioavailability. One of these problems is the ineptitude to keep the dosage form in the specific region of the gastrointestinal tract. Drug absorption from the gastrointestinal tract is a complicated process and is referred to several variables (Dey, et al., 2008). It is generally recognized that the proportion of gastrointestinal tract drug absorption is related to contact time with the small intestinal mucosa. Hence, small intestinal transit time is a salient characteristic for drugs that are not completely absorbed. General human physiology including the details of gastric emptying, motility patterns, and physiological and formulation variables influencing the celestial emptying are explained to understand gastric retention and floating drug delivery systems (Kar, et al., 2015). Gastro retentive systems can reside in the gastric part for many hours and thus remarkably enhance the gastric residence time of drugs. Better bioavailability, less drug wastage and, improved solubility of drugs that are less soluble in a high pH environment are the results of prolonged gastric retention. Local drug delivery to the stomach and proximal small intestines are also the applications of prolonged gastric retention. Gastro retention results in providing increased bioavailability of new products having new therapeutic properties and remarkable uses for patients. Mechanisms that help provide controlled gastric retention of solid dosage forms include flotation, mucoadhesion, sedimentation, expansion, modified shape systems, or, through the contemporaneous administration of pharmacological factors that prolong gastric emptying (Arora, et al., 2005; Sharma, et al., 2011).

Short gastric residence time and unpredictable gastric emptying rate are the two complications faced by orally administered controlled release dosage forms (Arora, et al., 2005; Sharma, et al., 2011).

The basic mechanism of floatation is followed to attain gastric retention for developing floating drug delivery systems (FDDS). It is observed that variation in gastric physiology (such as gastric pH, motility) show both intra-as well as inter-subject variance exhibiting notable influence on gastric retention time and drug delivery pattern. The latest developments of FDDS involving the physiological and formulation variables affecting gastric retention approaches to increase gastric retention time and their classification are covered briefly. The studies to evaluate the performance and applications of floating systems are also highlighted (Shah, et al., 2009).

5.1.1 Factors Affecting Gastric Retention

Several factors affecting the efficacy such as the gastro-retentive system, control the gastric retention time (GRT) of the dosage form. Some of these factors are mentioned below.

a) Density: GRT being a function of dosage form buoyancy, is dependent on the density.

b) Size: Dosage form units having a diameter of more than 9.5 mm are reported to have an enhanced GRT.

c) The shape of dosage form: Tetrahedron and ring-shaped devices having the flexural modulus of 48 and 22.5 kilopounds per square inch are reported to possess better GRT.

d) Single or multiple unit formulation: Multiple unit formulations predict better release profile and minor impairing of action due to abortion of units, help co-management of units having different release profiles or possessing agents and, exhibit a greater extent of safety against dosage form failure as compared to single unit dosage forms.

e) Fed or unfed state: Strong motor activity or the migrating myoelectric complex (MMC) occur every 1.5 to 2 hr is the characteristic of the GI motility during fasting conditions. The MMC pushes undigested material from the stomach to the intestine and the GRT of the unit can be expected to be very short if the administration of the formulation matches with that of the MMC. Whereas, in the fed state, MMC is prolonged and GRT is remarkably longer.

f) Nature of the meal: Indigestible polymers or fatty acid salts lead the motility pattern of the stomach to the fed state, hence decreasing the gastric emptying rate and extending the drug release.

g) Caloric content: A meal high in proteins and fats can increase GRT from 4 to 10 hr.

h) Frequency of feed: when successive meals are given, due to the low frequency of MMC, the GRT can be increased by 400 minutes as compared to the single meal.

i) Gender: Mean ambulatory GRT in males (3.4 ± 0.6 hr) is rarely compared with their age and race-matched female counterpart (4.6 ± 1.2 hr), notwithstanding the weight, height and, body surface.

j) Age: people above the age of 70 have a remarkably longer GRT.

k) Posture: GRT can vary between the supine and upright ambulatory states of the patients.

l) Concurrent drug administration: Anticholinergics and opiates increase gastric emptying.

m) Biological factors: diabetes and Crohn's disease also affect GRT (Tripathi, et al., 2019; Dixit, 2011).

5.2 Principle of FDDS

Floating systems or hydro-dynamically controlled systems have low density and adequate buoyancy to float over the gastric agents and remain buoyant in the stomach without disturbing the gastric emptying rate for a prolonged time. The system keeps on floating on the gastric contents and gradually the drug is released at the desired rate from the system. After the drug is released completely, the residual system is emptied from the stomach. As a result, an increase in GRT and better regulation of the fluctuations in plasma drug concentration is achieved. However, apart from the minimum gastric content required to achieve the proper buoyancy retention principle, a minimum level of floating force (F) is also needed to keep the dosage form feasibly buoyant on the surface of the chyme. Based on granules, powders, capsules, tablets, laminated films and, hollow microspheres, many buoyant systems have been developed (Kotreka and Adeyeye, 2011).

Several approaches and strategies have been utilized to increase the retention of an oral dosage form in the stomach including floating systems, bioadgesive systems, swelling and expanding systems, high-density systems, and modified systems (Badoni, et al., 2012).

5.3 Classification of FDDS

FDDS is also defined as the hydro-dynamically balanced system (HBS). The bulk density of FDDS is less than the gastric fluids and so they are buoyant in the stomach without influencing gastric emptying rate for a longer time. The drug is released slowly at the desired rate from the system while the system is floating on the gastric contents. The residual system, after releasing the drug, is emptied from the stomach, ultimately increasing the GRT and better control of the fluctuations in plasma drug concentration (Singh and Kim, 2000). This delivery system is further divided into non-effervescent and effervescent (gas-generating system).

5.3.1 Non-Effervescent Systems

5.3.1.1 Colloidal Gel Barrier Systems

Hydrodynamically balanced system (HBS), thas has drugs with gel-forming hydrocolloids, was first manufactured by Sheth and Tossounian in 1975. These systems integrate a high level (20-75% w/w) of one or more gel-forming, highly swellable, cellulose-type hydrocolloids, polysaccharides and, matrix-forming polymers. The hydrocolloids in the system hydrate and develop a colloidal gel barrier surrounding its surface. The gel barrier monitors the rate of fluid penetration into the device and the ultimate release of the drug (Bahadur, et al., 2020).

5.3.1.2 Micro Porous Compartment Systems

The base of this technique is the encapsulation of a drug reservoir inside a microporous chamber with perforations along its top and bottom walls. To avoid any direct contact of the gastric mucosal surface with the undissolved drug, the peripheral walls of the drug reservoir chamber are completely secured (Lodh, et al., 2020).

5.3.1.3 Multiparticulate System

Comprising of a multiplicity of small discrete units, floating beads multi-particulate drug delivery systems are oral dosage forms, where each unit exhibits some distinct properties. The dosage form of the drug substances, in these systems, are divided on a plurality of the subunit, generally made up of thousands of spherical particles having a diameter ranging from 0.05-2.00 mm. Hence, the active substance in multi particulate dosage forms is present in form of many small independent subunits, making feasible pharmaceutical formulations. These subunits are incorporated into a sachet to deliver the required total dose (Dey, et al., 2008).

5.3.1.4 Microballoons

Various approaches are utilized to deliver substances at the target site in a controlled release manner. One of such approaches is to use polymeric microballoons as a carrier for drugs. Hollow microspheres are defined as microballoons. When immersed in aqueous media, microballoons floated *in vitro* for 12 hours. Radio graphical studies showed that on oral administration to humans, microballoons were dispersed in the upper part of the stomach and remained there for three hours against peristaltic movements (Ayre, et al., 2016; Kumar, et al., 2016).

5.3.2 Effervescent Systems

The incorporation of a floating chamber that may be filled with vacuum, air or inert gas, can be used to make a delivery system float in the stomach (Daraee, et al., 2016).

5.3.2.1 Volatile Liquid Containing Systems

These systems possess an inflatable chamber that has a liquid e.g. ether, cyclopentane, that gasifies at body temperature to stimulate the inflation of the chamber in the stomach. There are two chambers in this system; one contains drugs and the other contains volatile liquid. Containing a hollow deformable unit, these systems are osmotically controlled floating systems (Gadge, et al., 2019; Jassal, et al., 2015; Hafeez, et al., 2013).

a) Intra-gastric floating gastrointestinal drug delivery systems: Vacuum, air, or a non-toxic gas-filled chamber causes floatation in these systems. While, inside a microporous compartment, the drug reservoir is encapsulated.

b) Inflatable gastrointestinal delivery systems: An inflatable chamber containing liquid ether is incorporated in these systems. The ether later gasifies at body temperature and flattens the chamber in the stomach.

c) Intra-gastric osmotically controlled drug delivery systems: In these systems, an osmotic pressure controlled drug delivery device and an inflatable floating aid is entrapped in a biodegradable capsule. In the stomach, the capsule immediately disintegrates to liberate the intra-gastric osmotically controlled drug delivery apparatus.

5.3.2.2 Gas generating systems

The effervescent reaction between carbonate/bicarbonate salts and citric/tartaric acid to liberate CO_2, that gets trapped in the jellified hydrocolloid layer of the system is utilized by these buoyant systems, thus reducing its specific gravity and making it float over chyme. A multiple-unit type of floating pills that produce CO_2 has also been manufactured. The system contains a sustained-release pill as the seed, covered by double layers. The core layer is an effervescent layer comprising sodium bicarbonate and tartaric acid. The outer layer containing PVA, shellac, etc., is a swell able membrane. Another effervescent system containing a telescopic spring, that controls the drug release from the polymer matrix, has also been formed. The general approach for developing these systems is resin beads incorporated with bicarbonate and glazed with ethyl cellulose. The glaze which is insoluble but permeable helps the permeation of water. Hence, carbon dioxide is liberated causing the beads to float in the stomach (Ghule, et al., 2014).

Intra-gastric single layer floating tablets or hydro-dynamically balanced systems (HBS): These are manufactured by considerably mixing the CO_2-producing agents and drug present inside the matrix tablet. They remain floating in the stomach not disturbing the gastric emptying rate for a long period.

Intra-gastric bilayer floating tablets: Comprising two layers of immediate release and sustained release respectively, these are also compressed tablets.

Multiple-unit type floating pills: These systems contain sustained-release pills as 'seeds' covered by two layers. Effervescent agents are present in the inner layer while the outer layer is the swell able membrane. When the system is submerged into the dissolution medium at the body temperature, it plunges at once and develops balloon-like swollen pills which float as they have lower density due to the production and entanglement of CO_2 (Hafeez et al., 2013; Nayak et al., 2013).

5.4 Advantages of FDDS

a) The gastro-retentive systems are beneficial for drugs absorbed through the stomach. E.g. ferrous salts, antacids.

b) Acidic drugs like aspirin cause irritation on stomach mucosa; hence, HBS formulation may be advantageous for the intake of aspirin and other similar drugs.

c) Intake of prolonged-release floating dosage forms, tablets or capsules, will lead to the dissolution of the drug in the gastric fluid and would be available for absorption in the small intestine after emptying of stomach contents. It is, therefore, anticipated that a drug will be completely absorbed from floating dosage forms if it resides in the solution form despite of the alkaline pH of the intestine.

d) Gastro-retentive systems are useful for drugs required for local action in the stomach e.g. antacids.

e) When there sturdy intestinal movement and a short transport time as might happen in a certain type of diarrhea, poor absorption is anticipated. Under such conditions, it would be beneficial to keep the drug floating in the stomach to get a relatively better outcome.

5.5 Disadvantages of FDDS

a) This system is not suitable for drugs having solubility or stability issues in GIT.

b) A high level of fluid in the stomach is required for the drug to float and work efficiently.

c) The only desirable candidates are those drugs that are absorbed throughout GIT and undergo distinct first-pass metabolism.

d) Some drugs present in the floating system can also irritate the gastric wall.

5.6 Evaluation Parameters of FDDS

Various studies have reported in the literature that pharmaceutical dosage forms showing gastric residence *in vitro* floating behavior exhibit prolonged gastric residence *in vivo* (Schneider, et al., 2019).

5.6.1 Pre-Compression Parameters

Bulk density, tapped density, compressibility index (Carr's index), Hausner's ratio, angle of repose, and drug excipient interaction are some of the main pre-compression parameters that impact the floating drug delivery systems (Shaikh, et al., 2018).

5.6.2 Compression Parameters

In the case of tablets, hardness, friability, assay, and content uniformity are used for evaluation. Tablet density and weight variation, swelling indices, floating lag time and total floating time were also determined (Tadros, 2010). *In vitro,* drug release studies are also performed (Gohel, et al., 2004). Drug loading, drug entrapment efficiency, particle size analysis, surface characterization, micromeritic studies and percentage yield are some of the key parameters affecting the characteristics of FDDS (Jain, et al., 2005). Pharmacokinetic studies are also performed for evaluating FDDS (Thakar, et al., 2013).

5.7 Applications of FDDS

5.7.1 Enhanced Bioavailability

The bioavailability of riboflavin CR-GRDF (controlled release-gastro retentive drug formulation) is remarkably increased as compared to the administration of non-GRDF controlled release polymeric formulations (Garg and Gupta, 2008; Manish and Hardik, 2013).

5.7.2 Sustained Drug Delivery

Orally administered controlled release formulations have limitations such as short gastric residence time in GIT. These problems can be managed by HBS systems that can reside in the stomach for the prolonged time (Soni, et al., 2018).

5.7.3 Site-Specific Drug Delivery Systems

These systems are specifically utilized for drugs that are particularly absorbed from the stomach or the proximal part of the small intestine. This minimizes the side effects that are caused by the drug in the blood circulation. Furthermore, dosing frequency is also reduced due to prolonged gastric availability from a site-directed delivery system (Stillhart et al., 2020).

5.7.4 Absorption Enhancement

Potential candidates to be formulated as FDDS are the drugs that have poor bioavailability due to site-specific absorption from the upper part of the GIT, thus increasing the absorption to maximum (Niharika, et al., 2018).

5.7.5 Reduced Toxic Effects at Colon

The toxic effects of the drug on the colon are reduced due to the retention of the drug in the stomach in the HBS systems. Hence, unwanted activities of drugs e.g. resistance caused by beta-lactam antibodies can be prevented in the colon (Garg and Gupta, 2008).

5.7.6 Reduced Fluctuations of Drug Concentration

Regular intake of the gastro retentive drug formulations develops blood drug concentrations within a narrow range as compared to the immediate release dosage forms. Hence, concentration-dependent adverse effects that are linked with peak concentrations can be avoided because the fluctuations in drug effects are minimized (Bhandwalkar, et al., 2020).

5.8 References

Arora, S., Ali, J., Ahuja, A., Khar, R. K., & Baboota, S. (2005). Floating drug delivery systems: a review. Aaps PharmSciTech, 6(3), E372-E390.

Ayre, A., Dand, N., & Lalitha, K. G. (2016). Gastro-retentive floating and mucoadhesive drug delivery systems-insights and current applications. IOSR J Pharma and Bio Sci, 11(3), 89-96.

Badoni, A., Ojha, A., Gnanarajan, G., & Kothiyal, P. (2012). Review on gastro retentive drug delivery system. The pharma innovation, 1(8, Part A), 32.

Bahadur, S., Manisha, S., Baghel, P., Yadu, K., & Naurange, T. (2020). An overview on various types of gastroretentive drug delivery system. ScienceRise: Pharmaceutical Science, (6 (28)), 4-13.

Bhandwalkar, M. J., Dubal, P. S., Tupe, A. K., & Mandrupkar, S. N. (2020). Review on gastroretentive drug delivery system. Asian Journal of Pharmaceutical and Clinical Research, 38-45.

Daraee, H., Etemadi, A., Kouhi, M., Alimirzalu, S., & Akbarzadeh, A. (2016). Application of liposomes in medicine and drug delivery. Artificial cells, nanomedicine, and biotechnology, 44(1), 381-391.

Dey, N. S., Majumdar, S., & Rao, M. E. B. (2008). Multiparticulate drug delivery systems for controlled release. Tropical journal of pharmaceutical research, 7(3), 1067-1075.

Dixit, N. (2011). Floating drug delivery system. Journal of current pharmaceutical research, 7(1), 6-20.

Gadge, G., Sabale, V., Khade, A., & Mahajan, U. (2019). Current approaches on gastro retentive drug delivery system: an overview. International Journal of Pharmacy Research & Technology, 9(2), 16-28.

Garg, R. G. D. G., & Gupta, G. D. (2008). Progress in controlled gastroretentive delivery systems. Tropical journal of pharmaceutical research, 7(3), 1055-1066.

Ghule, P. N., Deshmukh, A. S., & Mahajan, V. R. (2014). Floating drug delivery system (FDDS): an overview. Research Journal of Pharmaceutical Dosage Forms and Technology, 6(3), 174.

Gohel, M. C., Mehta, P. R., Dave, R. K., & Bariya, N. H. (2004). A more relevant dissolution method for evaluation of a floating drug delivery system. Dissolution technologies, 11, 22-26.

Hafeez, A., Maurya, A., Singh, J., Mittal, A., & Rana, L. (2013). An overview on floating microsphere: Gastro Retention floating drug delivery system (FDDS). The Journal of Phytopharmacology, 2(3), 1-12.

Jain, S. K., Awasthi, A. M., Jain, N. K., & Agrawal, G. P. (2005). Calcium silicate based microspheres of repaglinide for gastroretentive floating drug delivery: Preparation and *in vitro* characterization. Journal of controlled release, 107(2), 300-309.

Jassal, M., Nautiyal, U., Kundlas, J., & Singh, D. (2015). A review: Gastroretentive drug delivery system (grdds). Indian journal of pharmaceutical and biological research, 3(01), 82-92.

Kar, P., Jones, K. L., Horowitz, M., Chapman, M. J., & Deane, A. M. (2015). Measurement of gastric emptying in the critically ill. Clinical nutrition, 34(4), 557-564.

Kotreka, U., & Adeyeye, M. C. (2011). Gastroretentive floating drug-delivery systems: a critical review. Critical Reviews™ in Therapeutic Drug Carrier Systems, 28(1).

Kumar, R., Kamboj, S., Chandra, A., Gautam, P. K., & Sharma, V. K. (2016). Microballoons: An advance avenue for gastroretentive drug delivery system-A review. UKJ Pharm Biosci, 4, 19-30.

Lodh, H., Sheeba, F. R., Chourasia, P. K., Pardhe, H. A., & Pallavi, N. (2020). Floating Drug Delivery System: A Brief Review. Asian Journal of Pharmacy and Technology, 10(4), 255-264.

Manish, J., & Hardik, P. (2013). Gastro retentive floating drug delivery system: a review. IJPRBs, 2(2), 358-77.

Nayak, A. K., Das, B., & Maji, R. (2013). Gastroretentive hydrodynamically balanced systems of ofloxacin: *In vitro* evaluation. Saudi Pharmaceutical Journal, 21(1), 113-117.

Niharika, M.G., Krishnamoorthy, K., Akkala, M., 2018. Overview on floating drug delivery system. Int J App Pharm, 10(6), 65-71.

Schneider, F., Koziolek, M., & Weitschies, W. (2019). *In Vitro* and in vivo test methods for the evaluation of gastroretentive dosage forms. Pharmaceutics, 11(8), 416.

Shah, S. H., Patel, J. K., & Patel, N. V. (2009). Stomach specific floating drug delivery system: A review. Int J Pharm Tech Res, 1(3), 623-33.

Shaha, S. H., Patel, J. K., Pundarikakshudu, K., & Patel, N. V. (2009). An overview of a gastro-retentive floating drug delivery system. Asian journal of pharmaceutical sciences, 4(1), 65-80.

Shaikh, S. C., Dnyaneshwar, S., Bhusari, D. V., Jain, S., Kochar, P. P., & Vikram, N. S. (2018). Formulation and evaluation of Ibuprofen gastro-retentive floating tablets. Univ J Pharm Res, 3(4), 20-25.

Sharma, N., Agarwal, D., Gupta, M. K., & Khinchi, M. (2011). A comprehensive review on floating drug delivery system. International Journal of Research in Pharmaceutical and Biomedical Sciences, 2(2), 428-441.

Singh, B. N., & Kim, K. H. (2000). Floating drug delivery systems: an approach to oral controlled drug delivery via gastric retention. Journal of Controlled release, 63(3), 235-259.

Soni, S., Ram, V., & Verma, A. (2018). Updates on approaches to increase the residence time of drug in the stomach for site specific delivery: brief review. International Current Pharmaceutical Journal, 6(11), 81-91.

Stillhart, C., Vučićević, K., Augustijns, P., Basit, A. W., Batchelor, H., Flanagan, T. R., ... & Müllertz, A. (2020). Impact of gastrointestinal physiology on drug absorption in special populations—An UNGAP review. European Journal of Pharmaceutical Sciences, 147, 105280.

Tadros, M. I. (2010). Controlled-release effervescent floating matrix tablets of ciprofloxacin hydrochloride: Development, optimization and in vitro–in vivo evaluation in healthy human volunteers. European journal of pharmaceutics and biopharmaceutics, 74(2), 332-339.

Thakar, K., Joshi, G., Sawant, K.K., 2013. Bioavailability enhancement of baclofen by gastroretentive floating formulation: statistical optimization, in vitro and in vivo pharmacokinetic studies. Drug development and industrial pharmacy, 39, 880-888.

Tripathi, J., Thapa, P., Maharjan, R., Jeong, S.H., 2019. Current state and future perspectives on gastroretentive drug delivery systems. Pharmaceutics, 11, 193.

Whitehead, L., Fell, J., Collett, J., Sharma, H., Smith, A.-M., 1998. Floating dosage forms: an in vivo study demonstrating prolonged gastric retention. Journal of controlled release, 55, 3 12

6. ION-EXCHANGE RESIN

Arooj Khalid

6.1 Introduction

In the recent two decades, controlled drug delivery systems are gaining propulsion as it reduces dosage frequency and patient compliance. One of the most enchanting methods for modified drug delivery systems is the use of ion-exchange resins (IER). Ion exchange resonates have been widely used in various pharmaceutical formulations for several decennia. IER are insoluble polymers that contain acidic or basic functional groups and have an affinity to interchange counter ions within aqueous media. An Ion exchange resin has a resemblance with a small bead having a diameter ranging from 1-2 mm. It is yellowish or white and is fabricated from an organic polymer substrate backbone. Ion exchange is a reversible process in which ions are interchanged between solid and liquid when an encounter a highly insoluble body. By the drug diffusion process, the drug is released from resinate after exchanging ions in the GI tract. In some cases, due to the high molecular weight of resins, they are unable to be absorbed from the body and hence termed inert (Srikanth, et al., 2010).

6.2 Structure and Chemistry of Ion Exchange Resin

IER is poly-electrolytes that are insoluble polymers having ionizable groups that are distributed along the polymer backbone. The most commonly used resins in different formulations are cross-linked polystyrene and poly methacrylate polymers. When IER comes in contact with a fluid like water, ions in the fluid get interchange with polyelectrolytes counter ions and remove physically from the fluid. An ion-exchange resin is an electrically charged polymer where one ion is replaced with another (Atyabi, et al., 1996).

Apart from it, numerous functional groups have charge, only a few are commonly used for man-made IER includes;

a) -COOH, which is weakly ionized to COO^-
b) -SO$_3$H, which is strongly ionized to $-SO_3^-$
c) -NH$_2$ which weakly attracts protons to form NH_3^+
d) Secondary and tertiary amines that attract proton weakly
e) -NR$_3^+$, which has a strong permanent charge (R stands for some organic group)

All these groups are enough for the suitable selection of resin with either weak or strong positive or negative charge (Anand, et al., 2001).

6.3 Types of Ion Exchange Resins

There are two major classes of ion-exchange polymers which are given below

> 6.3.1   Cation exchange resin
> 6.3.1.1 Strong acid
> 6.3.1.2 Weak acid
> 6.3.2   Anion exchange resin
> 6.3.2.1 Strong base
> 6.3.2.2 Weak base

6.3.1 Cation Exchange Resin

It is positively charged and prepared by the process of copolymerization of styrene and divinylbenzene and sometimes sulfonic groups are launched to benzene rings. The mechanism of the cation exchange process can be represented by the following reaction:

$$R\text{-}ex^+ + C^+ \rightarrow R\text{-}C^+ + ex^+$$

Here, resin- presents a polymer with SO3- sites, that are available for adhering with exchangeable cation (ex+), and C^+ presents a cation in the surrounding solution getting interchanged.

Cation exchange resins are further classified into two groups which are discussed below:

6.3.1.1 Strong Acid Cation Exchange Resins

These resins chemically behave similarly to a strong acid. All these resins are ionized in both acid (R-SO_3H) and salt form of sulfonic acid group and can further convert into the corresponding acid by the following reaction:

$$2(R\text{-}SO_3H) + NiCl_2 \rightarrow (R\text{-}SO_4)Ni + 2HCl$$

The sodium and hydrogen forms of strong acid resins are highly dissociated, these ions can be easily exchanged over the entire pH range. As result, the exchange proportions of strong acid resins are independent of the solution pH (Luo, et al., 2018).

6.3.1.2 Weak Acid Cation Exchange Resins

These resins act the same as weak organic acids that can be dissociated easily. the solution pH is highly dependent on the dissociation of weak acid rein. A typical weak acid resin has a capacity below a pH of 6.0, which makes it not compatible with deionizing acid metal finishing wastewater.

6.3.2 Anion Exchange Resins

Anions have functional groups having a positive charge and can be prepared by first chlormethylating benzene rings of the styrene-divinylbenzene copolymer to get attached to CH_2Cl groups and then the resultant product reacts with tertiary amines such as triethylamine. The anion exchange is chemically presented by an equation:

$$R\text{-}ex^- + A^- \rightarrow R\text{-}A^- + ex^-$$

Where, R^+ presents a resin polymer with the number of sites that are available for binding to the exchangeable anion (ex-), and A- indicates cations that are exchanging in the surrounding solution.

Anion exchange resins are further divided into two groups which are discussed below:

6.3.2.1 Strong Base Anion Exchange Resins

Strong base resins are highly ionized and can be utilized over the whole pH range. These resins are used in the hydroxide (OH) form for water deionization. They will react with anions in solution and can convert an acid solution to pure water.

$$R\text{-}NH_3OH + HCl \rightarrow R\text{-}NH_3Cl + H_2O$$

Regeneration with concentrated sodium hydroxide (NaOH) converts the depleted resin to the OH form (Soyluoglu, et al., 2020)

6.3.2.2 Weak base anion exchange resins

Weak base resins are like weak acid resins in that the degree of ionization is strongly influenced by pH. Hence, weak base resins exhibit minimum exchange capacity above a pH of 7.0. The weak base resin does not have an OH ion form as does the strong base resin.

$$R\text{-}NH_2 + HCl \rightarrow R\text{-}NH_2Cl$$

As result, regeneration demands only to neutralize the absorbed. Low-cost weakly basic reagents such as ammonia (NH_3) or sodium carbonate can be employed.

A typical cation-exchange resin is formulated by the copolymerization of styrene and divinyl-benzene. Throughout the polymerization process, linear chains are formed in polystyrene and these become covalently bonded with one another by divinylbenzene cross-linkage. Then if the sulphuric acid is allowed to react with this copolymer, sulphonic acid groups are inaugurated into most of the benzene rings of the styrene-divinylbenzene polymer, and the final product formed is known as cation-exchange resin. A distinctive anion exchange resin is developed by first chloromethylating the benzene rings of the three-dimensional styrene-divinylbenzene copolymers to adhere – CH_2Cl groups and then the resultant product reacts with a tertiary amine, such as trimethylamine. This provides the chloride salt of strong-base exchangers (Zhenhua, et al., 1997)

6.4 Role of IER in Controlled Drug Delivery Systems

Dose dumping, high risk of toxicity is the major disadvantage of controlled release formulation. So the IER dosage forms are highly recommended due to their physic-chemical stability, inert nature, uniformity in size, drug retarding properties, and fewer chances of dose dumping, spherical shape assists coating and equilibrium driven reproducible drug release in the ionic environment. The drug resinates can also be used as a drug reservoir, from where the drug is released in hydrophilic polymer tablets. Drug molecules bound to resins are released by appropriately charged ions in the GI tract, by the process of diffusion of free drug molecules (Jeong, et al., 2008).

6.5 General Method of Preparation of IER

The prime step involved in the preparation of drug-resinates is to clarify resins carefully. The process of purification is done by repeatedly cycling between sodium and hydrogen forms with cation-exchanger or in the case of anionic exchangers, cycling is done between hydrogen and chloride forms. After that, all impurities are removed by washing with water. Moreover, drugs that are formulated into resinates, should have acidic or basic groups in their chemical structure having a biological half-life of 2 to 6 hr. As result, it will be better absorbed from the GI tract and will stable in gastric juice (Barbaro. P, et al., 2009; Singh, et al., 2007).

6.6 Advantages of ion exchange resins

a) It is free from local and systemic toxicities.

b) Economic and readily available.

c) High drug loading capacity.

d) Taste masking.

e) Can be formulated into different dosage forms like tablets, capsules, suspensions.

6.7 Disadvantages of IER

a) Dose dumping is the critical problem

b) Variability in diet, water intake, and intestinal content of an individual can affect the release rate of the drug.

c) The concentration of ions that are present in an area of administration directly affects the release rate.

6.8 Drug loading in IER

Drug loading is done in two ways which are given below:

6.8.1 Column Process

In this process, equilibrium is developed by eluting highly concentrated drug solution through a bed of column of resin

6.8.2 Batch Process

In this process, with a large volume of concentrated drug solution, the resin particles are mixed and adhering free and the un-associated drug is removed by washing and after that, it is air-dried (Elder, et al., 2005).

6.9 Characteristics of IER

6.9.1 Exchange Capacity

The number of ionic sites per unit weight or volume is referred to as exchange capacity. As wet resin is hydrated in nature, so the weight basis value (meq per g) is greater than the volume-based exchange capacity. Consequently, it limits the amount of drug to be absorbed in resin. Carboxylic acid resins that are acquired from acrylic acid polymers have a high capacity of an exchange than sulphonic acid so a high percentage of the drug can be loaded in carboxylic acid resins (Bajpai. et al., 2007).

6.9.2 Cross- Linkage

The degree of cross-linking is highly affected by the physical structure of the resin particles. For resins, having a low degree of cross-linking can get a considerable amount of water and can swell into a structure that is soft and gelatinous. However, for resins having high divinylbenzene content take up a small amount of water and consequently brittle.

6.9.3 Particle Size

The particle size of resin depends on the rate of ion-exchange reaction. By decreasing the particle size of resin, the time required for the reaction to reach equilibrium will be decreased with the surrounding medium.

6.9.4 Porosity and Swelling

The amount of cross-linking substances that are used in polymerization is highly affects the porosity of an ion-exchanger. The extent of swelling is highly dependent on the structure of the resin and as a result, can affect the release properties of drug resinates. The hydrophilic functional groups that are adhered to a polymeric matrix are directly affected by the amount of swelling and are inversely affected by the degree of divinylbenzene cross-linking present in the resin.

6.9.5 Available Capacity

The capacity of an ion-exchanger depends on the ability to take up exchangeable ions. So in the preparation of drug resonates, the actual capacity obtained is highly dependent on the availability of a functional group of the drug.

6.9.6 Acid-Base Strength

Resins containing sulfonic, phosphonic, or carboxylic acid exchange groups have pKa values of 1, 2-3, and 4-6, respectively and anionic exchangers are quaternary, tertiary, or secondary ammonium groups having pKa values greater than 13, 7-9, or 5-9, respectively. Moreover, the rate at which drug is released from resonates in the gastric fluid is highly influenced by the pKa value of the resin (Reichenberg, 1953).

6.9.7 Stability

The ion-exchangers are highly inert and at ordinary temperature, vinyl benzene cross-linked resins are resistant to decomposition through the chemical attack, but degeneration occurs in the presence of storage gamma-ray sources.

6.9.7 Purity and Toxicity

Before the usage of resin in formulations, resins are needed to be purified carefully.

6.9.8 Resins Selectivity for Counter Ions

The degree of sorption increases, firstly, with counter ion, apart from normal ionic bond having a functional group of an exchanger, also interacts through van der- Waal forces with the resin matrix. Secondly, the counterion is less affected by complex formation with its co-ion or nonexchanging ion and lastly, counter ion that prompts polarization highly (Zhenhua, et al., 1997).

6.10 Evaluation of Ion Exchange resins

6.10.1 *In Vitro* Evaluation

In vitro dissolution test is the most important tool for the proper control and evaluation of drug resinate preparations. Methods that are commonly used to test drug-resinates include the on-column and the batch exposure of the resinate to the simulated gastric and intestinal fluid. The USP dissolution methods are employed to maintain the fixed volume of solvent with sufficient solubility to approximate sink conditions (Dia, et al., 2009).

6.10.2 In Vivo Evaluation

In vivo evaluation, the bioavailability of drug from drug-resinate complexes depends on both transit of the particles through GI tract and drug release kinetics. Drug release can occur only through the replacement of the drug by another ion with the same charge. As the exchange is an equilibrium process, so it depends on the ionic constitution and volume of the body fluid. Besides, the release is not instantaneous, and the drug must diffuse through the resin from the internal exchange sites. Therefore, time of exposure and agitation play a prime role in drug release kinetics. Moreover, when the drug-resin complex comes in contact with the mouth, a little amount of the drug is released in the stomach due to high acid concentrations. Anionic exchange resins and the strong cation exchangers will release a small amount of drug in the stomach. Conversely, the drug attached to the weak acids is released faster in the stomach. The high pKa value of the resin leads towards the formation of un-dissociated acid in equilibrium (Atyabi, et al., 1996).

Stomach emptying having fine particles follow a first-order or distributional process. The neutral pH in the intestine keeps all the ionic sites ionized, and the process of exchange remains continuous. In the large intestine, due to fecal matter, low fluid content, poor absorption in the colon, the desorption from resins and absorption into the body becomes slow (Cuna, et al., 2001).

6.11 Applications of IER

6.11.1 Pharmaceutical Applications

6.11.1.1 Taste Masking

To mask the bitter taste of formulations, many challenges have been faced by pharmaceutical industries for pediatric and geriatric patients. By masking taste, improves patient compliance and increases product credibility in the market. Out of many taste-masking methods, ion-exchange resins are very inexpensive. So, previously some of the workers have been used carbomer to mask the unpleasant and nauseating effect of erythromycin and clarithromycin, by adsorbing carbopol and then encapsulating with hydroxypropyl methylcellulose phthalate (Suhagiya, et al., 2010).

6.11.1.2 Elimination of Polymorphism

Polymorphism is the ability of a drug substance to exist as two or more crystalline phases that have dissimilar arrangements and conformations of the molecules in the crystal lattice. Huge efforts have been made by different pharmaceutical industries to evaluate polymorphs to make them more stable and soluble. So, in ion exchange resins, resonates completely abolished the problem of polymorphism.

6.11.1.3 Improve the Dissolution of Poorly Soluble Drugs

Ion exchange resinate plays a prime role to increase the dissolution rate of the poorly soluble drug. As the rate of dissolution can be problematic after micronization, so these problems are solved by using the ion exchange resin approach.

6.11.1.4 Enhancing Stability

The drug resinate is more stable than the original drug. For example, vitamin B12 has short shelf life while its resinate has a shelf life of more than two years. Another example is nicotine, which discolors on exposure to air and light, while resinate is more stable than is used in the manufacturing of chewing gums and lozenges.

6.11.1.5 Improving Physical Characteristics

As physical properties majorly affect the stability of the solid or liquid formulations, so here, resinates play an important role by increasing the stability and shelf life of the product. For instance, nicotine is in liquid form but its resinate is a highly stable free-flowing solid. The resins have a uniform, macro reticular morphology, that boosts up the flowability of the formulation (Khan, 2012).

6.11.2 Drug Delivery Applications

6.11.2.1 Oral Drug Delivery

As the major disadvantage of sustained-release or extended-release dosage forms is dose dumping that results in increasing toxicity, so ion exchange resins have been used to retain drug properties and to prevent dose dumping. Because of the increased physicochemical properties, inert nature, uniform size, and spherical shape, ion exchange resins are widely used in drug delivery systems (Atyabi, et al., 1996).

6.11.2.2 Nasal Drug Delivery

A novel nasal formulation, in the form of nicotine-Amberlite resin complex powder, has been formulated to provide an extended plasma profile for smoking cessation. Amberlite IRP69 and Amberlite IR120 are the same cationic exchange materials having similar ion exchange capacity but, because of their smaller particle size range (10-150micron meter), Amberlite IRP69 had good flow properties and absorptive capacity than Amberlite IR120.

6.11.2.3 Transdermal Drug Delivery

IER is also used in the formulation of transdermal drug delivery systems. The release rates of ketoprofen from carbopol-based gel vehicles containing ion-exchange fibers. The fluctuations of the release rate of ketoprofen from vehicles were lower than that of simple gels. Apart of it, ions could increase the rate and extent of ketoprofen delivery (Jaskari, et al., 2000).

6.11.2.4 Ophthalmic Drug Delivery

IER is also an ophthalmic drug delivery system. For instance, Betoptic S is a sterile ophthalmic suspension and contains 0.25 % betaxolol hydrochloride. It is designated to lower elevated intraocular pressure. The drug resinate complex is formed when the positively charged drug is bound to a cation ion-exchange resin (Jani, et al., 1994)

6.12.3 Diagnostic and Therapeutic Applications

Synthetic and natural polysaccharides that are based on ion-exchange resins have been used in diagnostic applications. They also play an important role as adsorbents of toxins, antacids, and bile acid-binding agents. Ion exchange resins are widely used in the treatment of liver diseases, renal insufficiency, urolithic disease, and occupational skin disease. It also has application in the control of cholesterol and potassium ion levels (Vijay, et al., 2014).

6.13 References

Anand, V., Kandarapu, R., & Garg, S. (2001). Ion-exchange resins: carrying drug delivery forward. *Drug Discovery Today*, 6(17), 905-914.

Arooj Khalid

Atyabi, F., Sharma, H. L., Mohammad, H. A. H., & Fell, J. T. (1996). Controlled drug release from coated floating ion exchange resin beads. *Journal of controlled release, 42*(1), 25-28.

Bajpai, S. K., Bajpai, M., & Saxena, S. (2007). Ion exchange resins in drug delivery. *Ion Exchange and Solvent Extraction, A Series of Advances, 18.*

Barbaro, P., & Liguori, F. (2009). Ion exchange resins: catalyst recovery and recycle. *Chemical reviews, 109*(2), 515-529.

Cuna, M., Alonso, M. J., & Torres, D. (2001). Preparation and in vivo evaluation of mucoadhesive microparticles containing amoxycillin–resin complexes for drug delivery to the gastric mucosa. *European journal of pharmaceutics and biopharmaceutics, 51*(3), 199-205.

Dia, V. P., Wang, W., Oh, V. L., De Lumen, B. O., & De Mejia, E. G. (2009). Isolation, purification and characterisation of lunasin from defatted soybean flour and *in vitro* evaluation of its anti-inflammatory activity. *Food Chemistry, 114*(1), 108-115.

Elder, D. P. (2005). Pharmaceutical applications of ion-exchange resins. *Journal of Chemical Education, 82*(4), 575.

Jani, R., Gan, O., Ali, Y., Rodstrom, R., & Hancock, S. (1994). Ion exchange resins for ophthalmic delivery. *Journal of Ocular Pharmacology and Therapeutics, 10*(1), 57-67.

Jaskari, T., Vuorio, M., Kontturi, K., Urtti, A., Manzanares, J. A., & Hirvonen, J. (2000). Controlled transdermal iontophoresis by ion-exchange fiber. *Journal of controlled release, 67*(2-3), 179-190.

Jeong, S. H., & Park, K. (2008). Drug loading and release properties of ion-exchange resin complexes as a drug delivery matrix. *International journal of pharmaceutics, 361*(1-2), 26-32.

Khan, S. N. (2012). Therapeutic applications of ion exchange resins. In *Ion Exchange Technology II* (pp. 149-168). Springer, Dordrecht.

Luo, T., Abdu, S., & Wessling, M. (2018). Selectivity of ion exchange membranes: A review. *Journal of membrane science, 555*, 429-454.

Reichenberg, D. (1953). Properties of ion-exchange resins in relation to their structure. III. Kinetics of exchange. *Journal of the American Chemical Society, 75*(3), 589-597.

Singh, I., Rehni, A. K., Kalra, R., Joshi, G., Kumar, M., & Aboul-Enein, H. Y. (2007). Ion exchange resins: Drug delivery and therapeutic applications. *Fabad Journal of Pharmaceutical Sciences, 32*(2), 91.

Soyluoglu, M., Ersan, M. S., Ateia, M., & Karanfil, T. (2020). Removal of bromide from natural waters: Bromide-selective vs. conventional ion exchange resins. *Chemosphere, 238*, 124583.

Srikanth, M. V., Sunil, S. A., Rao, N. S., Uhumwangho, M. U., & Murthy, K. R. (2010). Ion-exchange resins as controlled drug delivery carriers. *Journal of Scientific Research, 2*(3), 597-597.

Suhagiya, V. K., Goyani, A. N., & Gupta, R. N. (2010). Taste masking by ion exchange resin and its new applications: A review. *Int J Pharm Sci Res, 1*(4), 22-37.

Vijay, S., & Dr, C. S. C. (2014). Ion exchange resins and their applications. *Journal of Drug Delivery & Therapeutics, 4*(4), 115-123.

Zhenhua, L., Qineng, P., & Guojie, L. (1997). Recent advance in controlled drug delivery by ion exchange polymers [J]. *Ion Exchange And Adsorption, 6*.

7. METHYLCELLULOSE GLUTARATE MATRICES

Muhammad Yasir Ali
Shahid Shah

7.1 Introduction

Methylcellulose glutarate is a chemically modified polymer obtained by reacting methylcellulose with glutaric anhydride. It was prepared and used in the fabrication of controlled release matrices of different active pharmaceutical ingredients (Ali, et al., 2011). In the following section, we will discuss about its preparation method, characterization, and further use for controlling the release of the drug.

7.2 Preparation

7.2.1 Reaction Conditions

1: 0.5 molar ratio of methylcellulose (MC) to glutaric anhydride (GA) was computed based on molecular weight and the number of free hydroxyl groups present in monomer units of methylcellulose. Both of these were dissolved in tetrahydrofuran (THF) taken in the round bottom flask of the rotary evaporator and allowed to react at 50 $^\circ$C and 60 rpm in experimental design. The reaction mixture was allowed to react for 12 hr, accompanied by the use of a chiller to condensate the evaporated THF.

7.2.2 Washing

After sufficient time has passed (12 hr), excess of THF was removed by using a vacuum evaporator, at < 40 °C. The product was washed for several times with THF to remove the un-reacted anhydride (Goldman, et al. 1961) and filtered using a fluted filtration technique for rapid filtration.

7.2.3 Grinding

The product was dried on glass slabs in diffused sunlight for at least one week. Chunks of the product were then crushed by using a specially designed 13000 rpm cutter mill, bearing a cold water jacket. The ground material was then passed through 40 mesh and the material retained was again subjected to crushing. In this manner, all the material was crushed and get in homogenized particle size.

7.3 Evaluation of Product

For the evaluation of the product, the following tests were performed.

7.3.1 TLC System Development

For the confirmation of the product, either synthesized or not, TLC was used.

7.3.1.1 Stationary Phase

Silica gel is the most commonly used adsorbent in TLC studies (Braithwaite, 2012). So for this purpose, prepared silica gel (60) plates (20X20 cm) were used. Plates were cut to a suitable size (2X6 cm).

7.3.1.2 Sample Preparation and Spotting

MC, GA, and MCG were taken in separate test tubes and were dissolved in Ethanol: Water (9:1) solution. Sample spots were marked and samples were applied on TLC plates using capillary tubes and dried (at room temperature).

7.3.1.3 Mobile Phase Preparation

Mobile phases were prepared using Methanol and Chloroform (1:1, 3:2, and 2:3) and were taken in a TLC tank. The phase was then allowed to evaporate so that equilibrium is developed between the liquid mobile phase and its vapors in the air present above the liquid surface. Then this whole setup was checked to move the sample on the stationary phase to predetermined height.

7.3.1.4 Spot Location

After sufficient time has been passed (the mobile phase has moved up enough), plates were removed from the tank and air-dried.

The two most commonly used methods for the location of spots are (Watson, 1999);

- Ultraviolet light

- Location agents (e.g. Iodine Vapors)

During the present studies, both methods were employed.

7.3.1.5 Result Interpretation

MC is a hydrophilic polymer of repeated glucose monomers, while GA moiety is hydrophobic in nature. When both of these were reacted, esterification of MC occurred. The resultant product was a little bit hydrophobic in nature as compared to MC. Now after the development of TLC, it was observed that all the three (MC, GA, and MCG) showed different locations of the spot (depending upon solvent system). When 1:1 (methanol: chloroform) was used spots of GA and MCG traveled to the maximum height leaving MC near the spot slightly near the baseline. In the second solvent system, 3:2 (CH_3OH: $CHCl_3$), GA, and MC.G were eluted to less height as compared to the previous one and MC moved more. However in the third one where the system was 2:3 (CH_3OH:

CHCl$_3$). In this case, spots of GA and MCG moved to maximum height leaving MC very near to the baseline (compare with the first one). As the polarity (Naser-ud-Din, 1992) of chloroform is very low as compared to methanol, so as the concentration of chloroform was increased from 2 to 3 parts the more hydrophobic sample goes on moving to the maximum height (Figure 7.1), whereas movement of MC was to less height, this is due to hydrophobic nature of the polymer because it is less soluble in methanol and more soluble in chloroform, so that by increasing the ratio of chloroform the movement of spot is more and of that of MC is to less extent. However, in the 1:1 solvent system, MC moved more than the last one (2:3).

In the presence of the same solvent system, samples were moved to some extent depending upon the polarity of the solvent and sample. The more polar system will move the more polar sample to maximum height and vice versa. The same was observed in this experiment. As in solvent system, the concentration of polar one (methanol) was increased MC moved to the height more as compared the system in which methanol was in less concentration. The reverse was observed in the case of less polar solvent (chloroform).

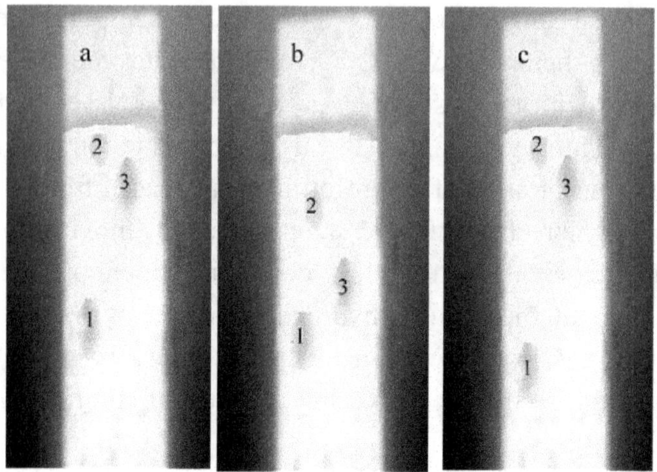

Figure 7.1: TLC in three different solvent systems: methanol: chloroform {1:1 (a), 3:2 (b) and 2:3 (c)}.

7.3.2 MALDI

Samples of reactant and product were evaluated by MALDI (Ultraflex TOF/TOF PRF-S02) using 1000 shots.

Different fragments depending upon the m/z values were being characterized. Two different peaks were observed first one at m/z 421.202 and the second one at m/z 727.010. This represents the loss of M^+-CH_3O, M^+-$C_5H_6O_3$, M^+-$C_6H_{12}O_6$, M^+-CH_3O-CH_3, M^+-$C_6H_{12}O_6$-CH_3O-CH_3, . All these can be represented as follows;

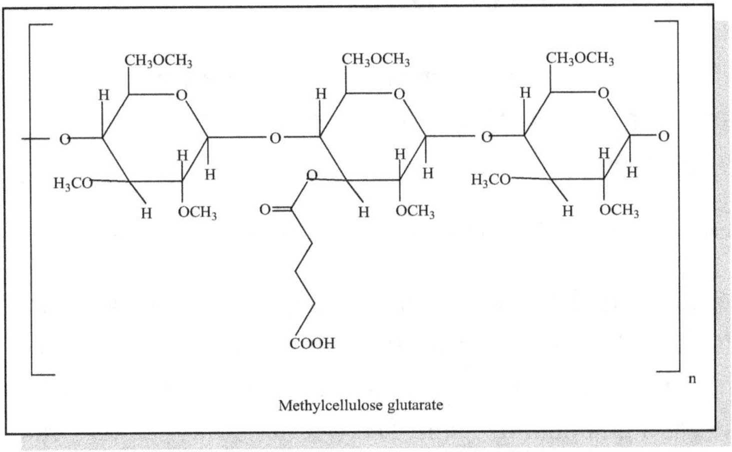

Figure 7.2: Proposed structure of Methylcellulose Glutarate.

7.3.4 Elemental Analysis

Samples subjected to the elemental analysis for the analysis of C, H, and O using Carlo Erba.

Samples subjected to the elemental analysis for the analysis of C, H, and O. Following table shows the percentage (%) of these elements;

Table 7.1: Elemental analysis of polymer.

Sample	% C	% H	% O
MC	48.662	7.521	41.820
MCG	47.474	6.882	43.264

7.4 Preparation of Matrices

MCG was used for the preparation of different formulations using Captopril (CPTL). The following method was used for this purpose.

7.4.1 Preparation of Granules (Wet Granulation)

All the materials were passed through sieve No. 40. CPTL, MCG, and Lactose were mixed thoroughly. 5 % solution of polyvinyl pyrrolidine (PVP) in isopropyl alcohol (IPA) was used as a granulating agent. The wet mass was passed through 20 mesh and air-dried for 24 hr to completely evaporate IPA.

7.4.2 Compression

Mg Stearate was mixed with granules thoroughly as a lubricant. The weight of granules was adjusted (308.5 mg) and tablets were compressed using a single punch machine at constant adjusted force. Formulations from F.I to F.V prepared. Each tablet consists of CPTL (50 mg), MCG (50-250 mg), lactose (50-200), povidone (8 mg) and Mg stearate (0.5 mg).

Table 7.2: Different formulations of Captopril (CPTL) using Methylcellulose Glutarate (MCG) as release modifier.

Codes	CPTL (mg)	MCG (mg)	Lactose (mg)
F.I	50	50	200
F.II	50	100	150
F.III	50	150	100
F.IV	50	200	50
F.V	50	250	-

7.6 *In Vitro* Evaluation of Matrices

The *in vitro* dissolution of all the capsules was determined using the USP apparatus II, paddle method (Pharma Test 903085, Germany). The test was performed in 900 ml distilled water as the dissolution medium with the temperature maintained at 37.0 ± 0.5 °C, while the stirring speed was set at 50 rpm. A sample of about 5 ml each was collected at 0.5, 1, 1.5, 2, 3, 4, 6, 8, 10, and 12 hr with an auto-sampler (Pharma Test PTFC II, Germany) after filtering through millipore filters. At the end of 12 hr the matrix was pressed in the dissolution vessels to obtain homogeneous dispersion and the stirring continued for another 15 min. Samples were then collected and analyzed for drug content. The final reading represented the total amount of drug released and was used to determine the percentage of drug released at different sampling intervals. All the samples were analyzed directly at 275 nm for CPTL using a UV-spectrophotometer (IRMECO UV-VIS U2020). All the tests were run in triplicate and results were represented as triplicate.

Figure 7.3 represents the effect of polymer concentration on the CR release data of the matrix tablets. Different MCG concentrations were used to evaluate their effect on the CR of the tablets. At the lower amount of MCG almost 100 % of the drug was released within 6 hr while at higher concentration about 60 % of the drug was released during the same interval. Therefore, it seems that the time of dissolution is related to the amount of polymer used in the matrices and the dissolution time was increased with the increasing amount of MCG. When the matrix system contacted water as dissolution medium, there was no gelling of the polymer due to the inability of the polymer to accommodate water. Instead, the matrix system seemed to be disintegrated and dissolved completely after 8 hr. Moreover, all the formulations were also evaluated using different kinetic models.

7.7 Assessment of Drug Release Kinetics

Drug release kinetics is assumed to reflect different release mechanisms of the sustained release matrix system. Therefore, kinetic models including the zero-order release equation, Higuchi square equation and Korsmeyer model were applied to analyze the in vitro data to find the equation with the best fit (Aslam, et al., 2012; Farago, et al., 2008; Bravo, et al., 2004; Tahara, et al., 1995). For further detail, see section 4.4.2.1

It was seen that as the concentration of polymer was increased the system began to follow zero-order kinetics due to greater values of r compared to the values obtained from other models. Therefore, the formulation F.V was found to be the best fit in the zero-order release pattern. The result of this study was in good agreement with the reported studies of Hayashi, et al., (2005) and Khairuzzaman, et al., (2006). In the reported studies, HPMC was used to note the effect of its various concentrations in the release of aspirin and theophylline and the release pattern was found to follow the zero-order kinetics.

7.8 Effect of Different Testing Conditions on Drug Release Rate from Matrices

In addition to the release profile in the water, the selected formulations were also tested at three different pH values i.e. 0.1 N HCl and phosphate buffer (pH 4.0 and 7.0). The effect of stirring speed on release rate was also evaluated on the test matrix tablets. The different rotation speeds are 50, 75, and 100 rpm.

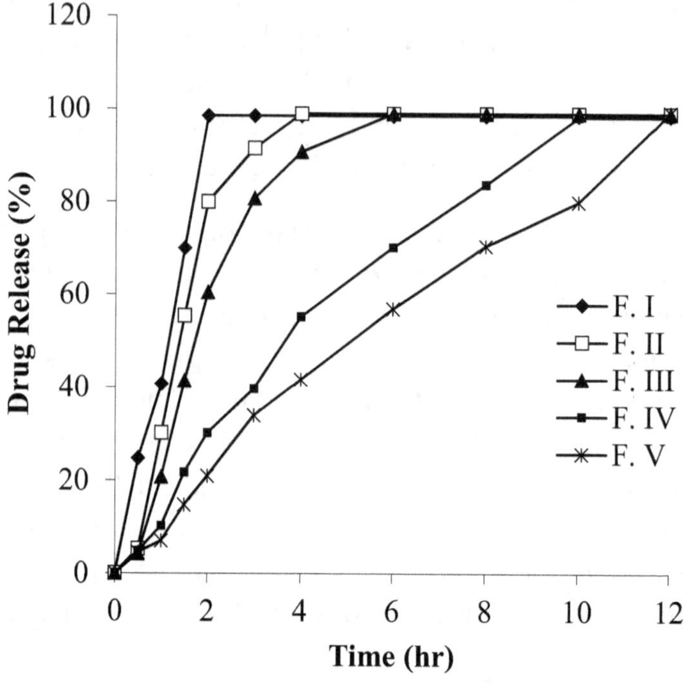

Figure 7.3: Influence of Methlycellulose Glutarate on *in vitro* release of Captopril.

7.8.1 Phosphate Buffer pH 4.0

This can be prepared by dissolving 6.8 g of potassium dihydrogen orthophosphate in 700 ml of water and then adjusting the pH, if necessary, with a 10 % v/v solution of orthophosphoric acid. The final volume is mad 1000 ml with water (BP, 2004).

7.8.2 Phosphate Buffer pH 7.0, Mixed

This can be prepared by dissolving 0.50 g of anhydrous disodium hydrogen orthophosphate and 0.301 g of potassium dihydrogen orthophosphate in sufficient water to produce 1000 ml (BP, 2004).

7.8.3 0.1 N HCl

The concentrated solution of HCl (35 %) was used to prepare 0.1N HCl solution.

Figure 7.4 shows the release profiles of CPTL from the selected formulation (F.V) at different pH values namely pH 7.0, pH 4.0, and 0.1 N HCl. The release profiles in water and in all other media were similar and more than 50 % in the first 4 hr of the sampling intervals.

Figure 7.5 shows the release profile of the selected formulation (F.V) at three different stirring speeds. As the stirring speed was increased, the disintegration of the test matrix was affected indicating erosion of the matrix at a faster rate. The percentage drug released was about 75%, 80 %, and 85 % at 50, 75, and 100 rpm respectively after 6 hr of sampling intervals. At higher stirring speed, complete dissolution took place within 8-10 hr while at 50 rpm it took 12 hr to release 100 % of the drug.

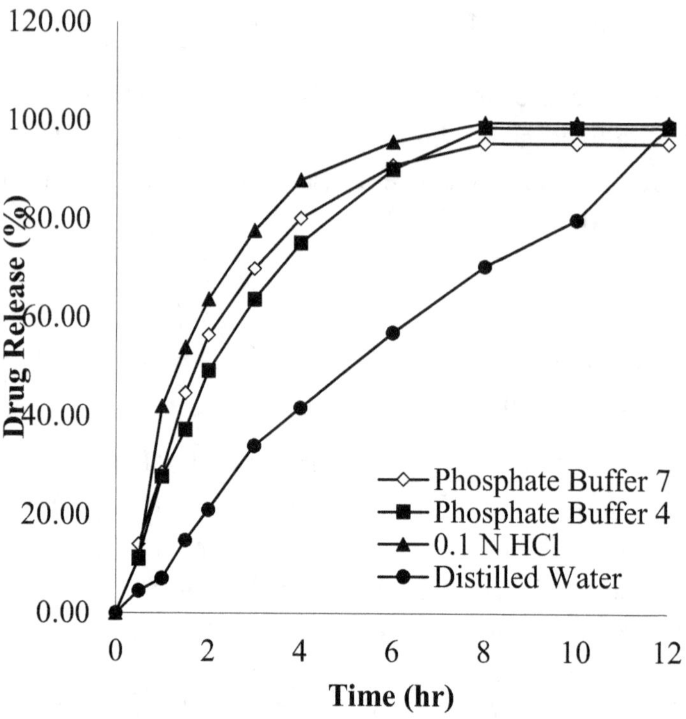

Figure 7.4: Influence of pH on *in vitro* release of Captopril from matrix tablet containing Captopril-Methylcellulose Glutarate in 1:5 ratio.

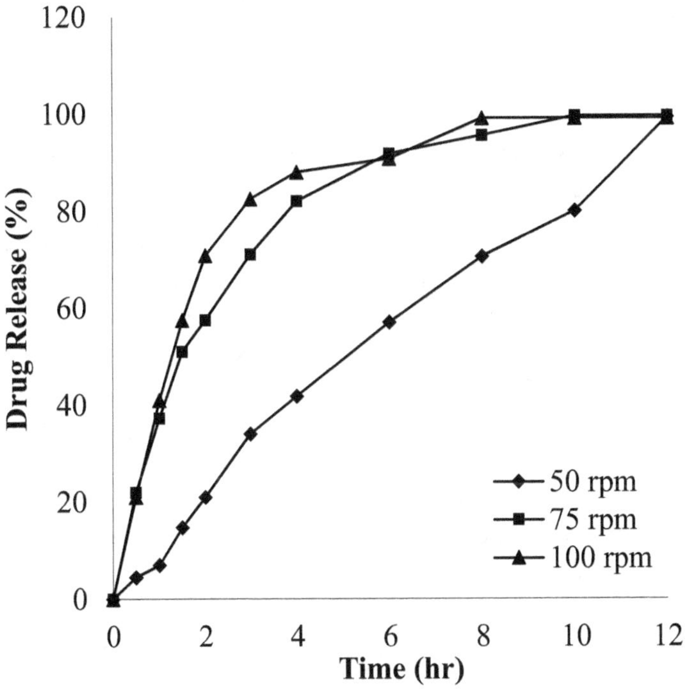

Figure 7.5: Influence of stirring speed on *in vitro* release of captopril from matrix tablet containing Captopril-Methylcellulose Glutarate in 1:5 ratio.

7.9 References

Ali, Y., Ahmed, S., & Ahmed, I. (2011). Sustained release of captopril from matrix tablet using methylcellulose in a new derivative form. *Lat. Am. J. Pharm*, *30*(9), 1696-1701.

Aslam, Z., Akhter, K. P., Ahmad, M., Aamir, M. N., Naeem, M., & Ali, M. Y. (2012). Preparation of modified-release tramadol tablets and drug release evaluation using dependent and independent modeling approaches. *Lat. Am. J. Pharm, 31*(10), 1417-21.

Braithwaite, A., & Smith, J. F. (2012). *Chromatographic methods.* Springer Science & Business Media.

Bravo, S. A., Lamas, M. C., & Salomon, C. J. (2004). Swellable matrices for the controlled-release of diclofenac sodium: Formulation and *in vitro* studies. *Pharmaceutical development and technology, 9*(1), 75-83.

Dr. Naser-ud-Din, Introduction of chromatography, 1992: 21.

Farago, P. V., Raffin, R. P., Pohlmann, A. R., Guterres, S. S., & Zawadzki, S. F. (2008). Physicochemical characterization of a hydrophilic model drug-loaded PHBV microparticles obtained by the double emulsion/solvent evaporation technique. *Journal of the Brazilian Chemical Society, 19*(7), 1298-1305.

Farago, P. V., Raffin, R. P., Pohlmann, A. R., Guterres, S. S., & Zawadzki, S. F. (2008). Physicochemical characterization of a hydrophilic model drug-loaded PHBV microparticles obtained by the double emulsion/solvent evaporation technique. *Journal of the Brazilian Chemical Society, 19*(7), 1298-1305.

Goldman, P., & Vagelos, P. R. (1961). The specificity of triglyceride synthesis from diglycerides in chicken adipose tissue. *Journal of Biological Chemistry, 236*(10), 2620-2623.

Hayashi, T., Kanbe, H., Okada, M., Suzuki, M., Ikeda, Y., Onuki, Y., ... & Sonobe, T. (2005). Formulation study and drug release mechanism of a new theophylline sustained-release preparation. *International journal of pharmaceutics, 304*(1-2), 91-101.

Khairuzzaman, A., Ahmed, S. U., Savva, M., & Patel, N. K. (2006). Zero-order release of aspirin, theophylline and atenolol in water from novel methylcellulose glutarate matrix tablets. *International Journal of Pharmaceutics*, *318*(1-2), 15-21.

Tahara, K., Yamamoto, K., & Nishihata, T. (1995). Overall mechanism behind matrix sustained release (SR) tablets prepared with hydroxypropyl methylcellulose 2910. *Journal of controlled release*, *35*(1), 59-66.

Watson, D. G. (1999). Pharmaceutical AnalysisA Textbook for Pharmacy Students and Pharmaceutical Chemists.

8. NIOSOMES

Daulat Haleem Khan

8.1 Introduction

Niosomes are non-ionic surfactant vesicles having the tendency to self-assemble and stabilized with the help of cholesterol with or without the addition of charge aiding ingredients. They are prepared as liposomes and are similar in physical characteristics. They are also unilamellar and multilamellar. They have more advantages over liposomes as they are easy to develop, surfactants can be derivatized with high versatility, and less costly to produce and preserve (Uchegbu & Florence, 1995).

The prominent features of niosomes that leads to their vast applications in pharmaceutical product development and cosmeceuticals are as below;

a) Niosomes can encapsulate hydrophilic and hydrophobic drugs in the same manner as liposomes.
b) They are osmotically stable and active.
c) Due to the presence of hydrophilic and hydrophobic components in the basic structure, they can encapsulate a wide range of drugs depending upon their solubility.

d) They can be designed upon the desired size and fluidity.

e) They can deliver the drug to the target site and its bioavailability can be improved.

f) Niosomes can allow attachment of functional ligands for targeted delivery.

g) They are also used to increase the bioavailability of the least soluble drugs (Puvvada, et al., 2013).

8.2 Structural Components of Niosomes

Niosomes are composed of non-ionic surfactants, cholesterol, and sometimes charge tailoring agents is indicated in Figure 8.1 (Moghassemi & Hadjizadeh, 2014).

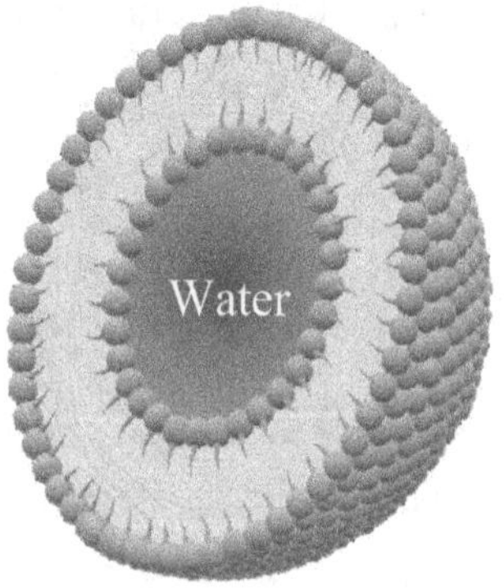

Figure 8.1: Structure of Niosome.

8.3 Classification of Non-Ionic Surfactants (General)

The non-ionic surfactants are neutral in nature and do not have a charge. When nonionic surfactants are dispersed in the aqueous phase the hydrophobic tails arrange themselves towards the organic phase (towards each other) and hydrophilic heads become oriented towards the aqueous phase (away from each other) (Abdelkader, et al., 2014). Non-ionic surfactants are used for the preparation of niosomes and they are classified as follows;

8.3.1 Alkyl Ethers

Alkyl ethers are further divided into two subclasses depending upon their hydrophilic heads, which are described as follows:

8.3.1.1 Alkyl Glycerol Ethers

These are the non-ionic surfactants having the glycerol subunits or the larger sugar molecule. These types of surfactants have been used to encapsulate anticancer drugs. Their behavior is to alter the pharmacokinetics of the drugs (Kuotsu, et al., 2010).

8.3.1.2 Alkyl Oxyethylene Ethers

These are the surfactants having repeated units of oxyethylene (Brij®). They have been used for the encapsulation of drugs for oral delivery to prevent the destructive effect of gastric acid.

They have been used, especially for the delivery of insulin (Pardakhty, et al., 2007).

8.3.1.3 Alkyl esters

These types of surfactants include sorbitan fatty acid esters (Span®) and polyoxyethylene fatty acid esters (tween®). They have been used in oral delivery of drugs, parenteral, topical, cosmeceuticals, and even in foodstuff preparation. The advantage of the usage of these surfactants are non-toxic and non-irritant (Muzzalupo, et al., 2011).

8.3.1.4 Pluronics

Pluronics are poly (ethylene oxide) and poly (propylene oxide) triblock copolymers. They have different numbers of ethylene oxide and propylene oxide units and due to which they have different HLB values. They have been used for the delivery of cytotoxic drugs. They have the capability to modify the drug response by making it targeted. Pluronics have the tendency to internalize the doxorubicin and other cytotoxic drugs for a longer duration of time by neutralization of the effect of P-glycoproteins and reduces the anticancer drug resistance. The solubility of poorly water-soluble drugs is increased by using a pluronic class of amphiphiles (Alexander, et al., 2002).

8.3.1.5 Cholesterol

The effect of cholesterol on the niosomal formulation is also important. It affects the physical characters of the niosomes including their shape due to the interaction between cholesterol and non-ionic surfactants. Cholesterol (30 % to 50 %) is required for vesicular formation. The quantity of cholesterol needed for the development of niosomes is also dependent on the HLB value of the surfactant. When the HLB value increases from 10, more quantity of cholesterol is required. Some studies suggested that the entrapment efficiency of the drug is also dependent on the quantity of cholesterol. The presence of cholesterol provides mechanical and hydrodynamic stability to the niosomes. The role of cholesterol is controversial, some studies suggested that less amount of cholesterol along with span 60 results in high entrapment efficiency. The amount of cholesterol to be added in the formulation must be evaluated case by case, depending upon the nature of the non-ionic surfactant and model drug used (Marianecci, et al., 2014).

8.3.1.6 Charge Aiding Molecules

The niosomes can be stabilized by the addition of charge aiding molecules to the bilayer structure. The negative charge is given to the niosome by phosphatidic acid and dicetylphosphate. Similarly, stearylamine (SA) and cetylpyridinium oxide are used to give positive charge to niosomes. Due to these charge-inducing molecules niosomes do not aggregate due to repulsive forces. The niosomes labeled with a positive charge (SA) were used to encapsulate negatively charged polynucleotide with resulted in efficient transfection into cells. Charge aiding agents are used to make the less aggregating niosomes, to prolong the plasma circulation half-life of the vesicles of niosomes and the residence time of ocular surfactant vesicles are also prolonged. The concentration of charge aiding molecule between 2.5-5 mol % results in results in stable and discrete niosomes and higher concentration results in inhibition of niosomal vesicular formation. The zeta (ζ)-potentials over 30 mV results in stable niosomes due to least aggregation. The benefit of designing charged niosomes is to make the vesicles stable and with high percentage entrapment efficiency (% EE) and skin permeation (Pardakhty, et al., 2012).

8.4 Method of Preparation

Niosomes are used to encapsulate a wide variety of drugs and biotechnological products to deliver at the targeted site. For the manufacturing of niosomes, few methods are described as follows;

8.4.1 Thin Film Hydration Technique (TFH)

This is the simplest and extensively used method for the preparation of niosomes. In this method, non-ionic surfactant and cholesterol are dissolved in an organic solvent in a round bottom flask. The solution is then evaporated under a vacuum in a rotary evaporator to prepare the thin film by removing the organic solvent. The buffer (phosphate buffer saline) containing the drug is then introduced in the round bottom flask containing thin film to make it hydrated. The solution is then heated above the phase transition temperature of the surfactant which results in vesicular formation. The schematic flow diagram of thin-film hydration technique is shown in Figure 8.2 (Moghassemi & Hadjizadeh, 2014).

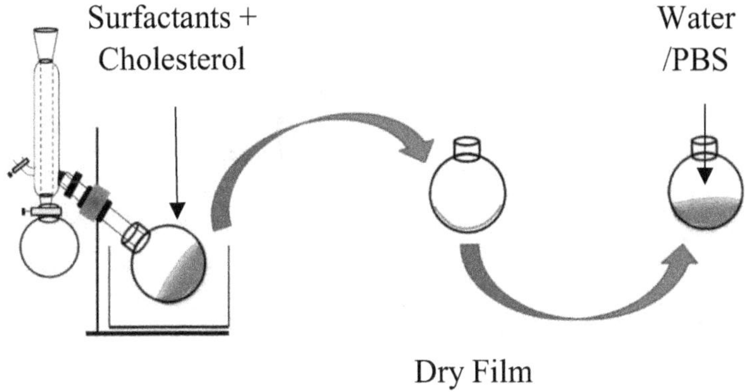

Figure 8.2: Thin-film hydration technique.

8.4.2 Reverse Phase Evaporation (REV)

In this method, cholesterol and surfactants are dissolved in the organic phase. Then aqueous phase containing the drug is added to the organic phase and sonicated until an emulsion is formed followed by evaporation at 40-60 °C. This evaporation phase will continue until complete hydration is done and the organic solvent is completely evaporated. During the evaporation, niosome vesicles are produced. The schematic flow chart of the REV technique is shown in Figure 8.3 (Moghassemi & Hadjizadeh, 2014).

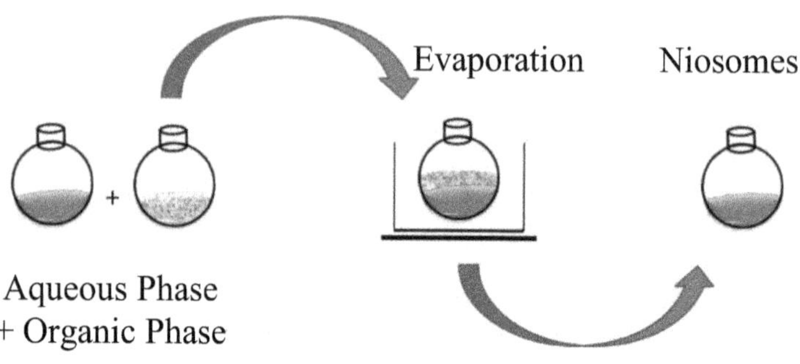

Figure 8.3: Reverse phase evaporation technique.

8.4.3 Ether Injection Method

In this method non-ionic surfactant, charge imparting agent, and cholesterol are dissolved in an organic solvent and this mixture is then injected into the aqueous drug solution at a temperature of 60 °C for the removal of solvent. This evaporation of solvents results in the formation of vesicles. The schematic flow protocol of the ether injection method is shown in Figure 8.4 (Moghassemi & Hadjizadeh, 2014).

8.4.4 Micro-Fluidization Method

In this method, the solution of surfactant and drug passed through an interaction chamber and then subjected to pass through cooling loop to eliminate the effect of heat during the interaction. The cooling of the resultant solution results in the formation of niosomal vesicles (Duncan, et al., 1997).

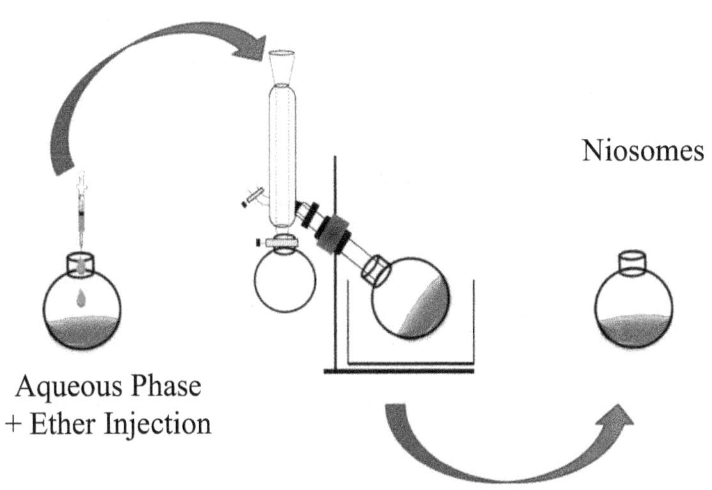

Figure 8.4: Ether injection method.

8.4.5 Trans-Membrane Method

In the trans-membrane method, the non-ionic surfactant and cholesterol are dissolved in an organic solvent and evaporated to make a thin film under reduced pressure. This thin film the hydrated with an acidic medium (citric acid) and vortexed. The obtained solution then freeze-thawed and then drug-containing solution added. The pH of the resultant is adjusted to 7.4 with the addition of disodium hydrogen phosphate (Baillie, et al., 1985).

8.4.6 Super-Critical Fluid Method

In this method, non-ionic surfactant and cholesterol are dissolved in an organic solvent and this solution is sent to view cell. The temperature of the cell raised to 60°C and 200bar pressure with carbon dioxide. This mixture is subjected to stirring with a magnet for 30 min. after mixing the pressure is released and niosomal dispersion is collected (Manosroi, et al., 2008a).

8.4.7 Bubble Method

In this method, amphiphilic surfactant, cholesterol, and phosphate buffer saline are added to the glass reactor having three necks. In one neck thermometer is inserted to check the temperature. In the second nitrogen gas was purged and in the third neck cooled waster was passed. The ingredients of the formulation were heated at 70°C, homogenized at the high shear rate for 15 min, and purged with nitrogen by bubbling resulted in niosome formation (Verma, et al., 2010).

8.4.8 Membrane Contactor

In this method, two-chamber equipment is used in which Shirasu porous glass membrane is used. In this non-ionic surfactant dissolved in organic solvent introduced into the chamber and aqueous solution, drug was also introduced from another side. They passed from the membrane due to the introduction of pressure and resulted in niosome production (Pham, et al., 2012).

8.4.9 Microfluidic Hydrodynamic Focusing

In this method of manufacturing, surfactant, cholesterol, and charge-inducing agents are dissolved in an organic solvent and placed in a glass scintillation vial. The organic solvent is removed from the vial and thin film is obtained. Isopropyl alcohol is added to the vial and drug-containing PBS is also added for the re-hydration of the dried film in microfluidic devices and resulted in niosomal vesicular formation (Lo, et al., 2010).

8.4.10 Proniosomal Technology

In this technology, the precursors of niosomes are generated and after that, they are rehydrated with water and agitated. It results in the production of niosomes and are used to deliver a variety of drugs (Moghassemi & Hadjizadeh, 2014).

8.5 Characterizations

The characterization of niosomes is done usually by the following techniques;

a) Fourier Transform Infrared (FTIR) spectroscopy.
b) Differential Scanning Calorimetry (DSC)
c) Entrapment efficiency (EE)
d) Differential Light Scattering (DLS)
e) Transmission Electron Microscopy (TEM)
f) Stability Studies
g) Drug Release Studies

8.6 Applications of Niosomes

Niosomes can be used for the delivery of a range of active pharmaceutical ingredients; a few examples are as follows;

Class	Examples
Anti-inflammatory Drugs	a) Diclofenac diethylammonium (Mansorsoi, et al., 2008)
	b) Aceclofenac (Nasr, et al., 2008)
	c) Lornoxicam (Kumbhar, et al., 2013)
Cytotoxic Drugs	d) Doxorubicin (Uchegbu, et al., 1994)
	e) 5-Flurouracil (Paolino, et al., 2008)
	f) Vincristine sulfate

<table>
<tr><td></td><td>(Parthasarathi, et al., 1994)</td></tr>
<tr><td></td><td>g) Cisplatin (Yang et al., 2013)</td></tr>
<tr><td>Antiviral Drugs</td><td>h) Acyclovir
(Monavari, et al., 2014)</td></tr>
<tr><td></td><td>i) Genciclovir (Akhter et al., 2012)</td></tr>
<tr><td>Gene Delivery</td><td>j) pCMSEGFP plasmid
(Puras, et al., (2014)</td></tr>
<tr><td>Proteins and Peptides</td><td>k) Insulin
(Pardakhty, et al., (2007)</td></tr>
</table>

8.7 References

Abdelkader, H., Alani, A. W. G., & Alany, R. G. (2014). Recent advances in non-ionic surfactant vesicles (niosomes): self-assembly, fabrication, characterization, drug delivery applications and limitations. Drug Delivery, 21(2), 87–100.

Akhter, S., Kushwaha, S., Warsi, M. H., Anwar, M., Ahmad, M. Z., Ahmad, I., ... & Ahmad, F. J. (2012). Development and evaluation of nanosized niosomal dispersion for oral delivery of Ganciclovir. *Drug development and industrial pharmacy*, *38*(1), 84-92.

Alexander V. Kabanova , Elena V. Batrakova, V. Y. A. (2002). Pluronic block copolymers as novel polymer therapeutics for drug and gene delivery. Journal of Controlled Release, 82(1), 189–212.

Baillie, A. . J., Florence, A. T., Hume, L. R., Muirhead, G. . T., & Rogerson, A. (1985). The preparation and properties of niosomes-non-ionic surfactant vesicles. The Journal of Pharmacy and Pharmacology, 37(12), 863–868.

Cametti, C. (2008). Polyion-induced aggregation of oppositely charged liposomes and charged colloidal particles: The many facets of complex formation in low-density colloidal systems. Chemistry and Physics of Lipids, 155(2), 63–73.

Duncan, R., Florence, A., Uchegbu, I., & Cociacinch, F. (1997). Drug Polymer conjugates encapsulated within niosomes.

Kumbhar, D., Wavikar, P., & Vavia, P. (2013). Niosomal gel of lornoxicam for topical delivery: in vitro assessment and pharmacodynamic activity. *AAPS pharmscitech, 14*(3), 1072-1082.

Kuotsu, K., Karim, K., Mandal, A., Biswas, N., Guha, A., Chatterjee, S., & Behera, M. (2010). Niosome: A future of targeted drug delivery systems. Journal of Advanced Pharmaceutical Technology & Research, 1(4), 374.

Lo, C. T., Jahn, A., Locascio, L. E., & Vreeland, W. N. (2010). Controlled self-assembly of monodisperse niosomes by microfluidic hydrodynamic focusing. Langmuir, 26(11), 8559–8566.

Manosroi, A., Jantrawut, P., & Manosroi, J. (2008). Anti-inflammatory activity of gel containing novel elastic niosomes entrapped with diclofenac diethylammonium. *International journal of pharmaceutics, 360*(1-2), 156-163.

Manosroi, A., Jantrawut, P., & Manosroi, J. (2008a). Anti-inflammatory activity of gel containing novel elastic niosomes entrapped with diclofenac diethylammonium. International Journal of Pharmaceutics, 360(1–2), 156–163.

Marianecci, C., Di Marzio, L., Rinaldi, F., Celia, C., Paolino, D., Alhaique, F., … Carafa, M. (2014). Niosomes from 80s to present: The state of the art. Advances in Colloid and Interface Science, 205, 187–206.

Moghassemi, S., & Hadjizadeh, A. (2014). Nano-niosomes as nanoscale drug delivery systems: An illustrated review. Journal of Controlled Release, 185(1), 22–36.

Monavari, S. H. (2014). The inhibitory effect of Acyclovir loaded nano-niosomes against herpes simplex virus type-1 in cell culture. *Medical journal of the Islamic Republic of Iran, 28*, 99.

Muzzalupo, R., Tavano, L., Cassano, R., Trombino, S., Ferrarelli, T., & Picci, N. (2011). A new approach for the evaluation of niosomes as effective transdermal drug delivery systems. European Journal of Pharmaceutics and Biopharmaceutics, 79(1), 28–

Nasr, M., Mansour, S., Mortada, N. D., & Elshamy, A. A. (2008). Vesicular aceclofenac systems: a comparative study between liposomes and niosomes. *Journal of microencapsulation, 25*(7), 499-512.

Oh, Y.-K., Kim, M. Y., Shin, J.-Y., Kim, T. W., Yun, M.-O., Yang, S. J., ... Choi, H.-G. (2006). Skin permeation of retinol in Tween 20-based deformable liposomes: in-vitro evaluation in human skin and keratinocyte models. Journal of Pharmacy and Pharmacology, 58(2), 161–166.

Paolino, D., Cosco, D., Muzzalupo, R., Trapasso, E., Picci, N., & Fresta, M. (2008). Innovative bola-surfactant niosomes as topical delivery systems of 5-fluorouracil for the treatment of skin cancer. *International journal of Pharmaceutics, 353*(1-2), 233-242.

Pardakhty, A., Shakibaie, M., Daneshvar, H., Khamesipour, A., Mohammadi-Khorsand, T., & Forootanfar, H. (2012). Preparation and evaluation of niosomes containing autoclaved Leishmania major: A preliminary study. Journal of Microencapsulation, 29(3), 219–224.

Pardakhty, A., Varshosaz, J., & Rouholamini, A. (2007). In vitro study of polyoxyethylene alkyl ether niosomes for delivery of insulin. *International journal of pharmaceutics, 328*(2), 130-141.

Pardakhty, A., Varshosaz, J., & Rouholamini, A. (2007). In vitro study of polyoxyethylene alkyl ether niosomes for delivery of insulin. International Journal of Pharmaceutics, 328(2), 130–141.

Parthasarathi, G., Udupa, N., Umadevi, P. I. L. L. A. I., & Pillai, G. (1994). Niosome encapsulated of vincristine sulfate: improved anticancer activity with reduced toxicity in mice. *Journal of drug targeting*, *2*(2), 173-182.

Pham, T. T., Jaafar-Maalej, C., Charcosset, C., & Fessi, H. (2012). Liposome and niosome preparation using a membrane contactor for scale-up. Colloids and Surfaces B: Biointerfaces, 94(1), 15–21.

Puras, G., Mashal, M., Zárate, J., Agirre, M., Ojeda, E., Grijalvo, S., ... & Pedraz, J. L. (2014). A novel cationic niosome formulation for gene delivery to the retina. *Journal of Controlled Release*, *174*, 27-36.

Puvvada, N., Rajput, S., Kumar, B. N. P., Mandal, M., & Pathak, A. (2013). Exploring the fluorescence switching phenomenon of curcumin encapsulated niosomes: In vitro real time monitoring of curcumin release to cancer cells. RSC Advances, 33(8), 2553–2557.

Uchegbu, I. F., & Florence, A. T. (1995). Non-ionic surfactant vesicles (niosomes): Physical and pharmaceutical chemistry. Advances in Colloid and Interface Science, 58(1), 1–55.

Uchegbu, I. F., Turton, J. A., Double, J. A., & Florence, A. T. (1994). Drug distribution and a pulmonary adverse effect of intraperitoneally administered doxorubicin niosomes in the mouse. *Biopharmaceutics & drug disposition*, *15*(8), 691-707.

Verma, S., Singh, S. K., Syan, N., Mathur, P., & Valecha, V. (2010). Nanoparticle vesicular systems: a versatile tool for drug delivery. J Chem Pharm Res, 2(2), 496–509.

Wu, I. Y., Bala, S., Škalko-Basnet, N., & Di Cagno, M. P. (2019). Interpreting non-linear drug diffusion data: Utilizing Korsmeyer-Peppas model to study drug release from liposomes. *European Journal of Pharmaceutical Sciences*, *138*, 105026.

Yang, H., Deng, A., Zhang, J., Wang, J., & Lu, B. (2013). Preparation, characterization and anticancer therapeutic efficacy of cisplatin-loaded niosomes. *Journal of microencapsulation*, *30*(3), 237-244